AF887431

Using Functional Genomics and Artificial Intelligence to Reverse Engineer Human Cancer Cells

Using Functional Genomics and Artificial Intelligence to Reverse Engineer Human Cancer Cells

By

Stephen P. Ethier

Cambridge Scholars Publishing

Using Functional Genomics and Artificial Intelligence to Reverse Engineer Human Cancer Cells

By Stephen P. Ethier

This book first published 2023

Cambridge Scholars Publishing

Lady Stephenson Library, Newcastle upon Tyne, NE6 2PA, UK

British Library Cataloguing in Publication Data
A catalogue record for this book is available from the British Library

Copyright © 2023 by Stephen P. Ethier

All rights for this book reserved. No part of this book may be reproduced, stored in a retrieval system, or transmitted, in any form or by any means, electronic, mechanical, photocopying, recording or otherwise, without the prior permission of the copyright owner.

ISBN (10): 1-5275-9230-8
ISBN (13): 978-1-5275-9230-8

TABLE OF CONTENTS

LIST OF ILLUSTRATIONS

LIST OF TABLES

PREFACE

My overriding motivation in writing this book is a phrase that you will encounter several times in the pages to come. That phrase is: "There is no cure for metastatic disease". The reason this phrase is so important is because, despite the enormous progress we have made over the decades from research on cancer, there has been very little progress for patients once their disease has spread to distant organs. And because of that, it is clearly time for us as a community to try some new approaches because standard chemotherapy, despite its uses in other phases of the disease, is not going to get us to the last mountaintop, the cure for metastatic cancer. In my opinion, one such strategy involves the application of modern artificial intelligence (AI) and machine learning (ML) methods to the mountains of genomic data that have been amassed from cancer patients and cancer-derived cell lines to develop strategies that can allow for truly personalized strategies for reverse engineering cancer in individual patients. The goal, therefore, of this book is to convince the reader that this is possible and, at the very least, an avenue worth pursuing. I should say at the outset that I will emphasize in this book how AI analysis of genomic data can lead us to better use of targeted cancer therapies. At the same time, other people are working on developing similar ways to use computational and AI methods to improve the use of immunotherapies for cancer, because immunotherapy provides another set of tools that can be used for patients with metastatic cancer. Since I am not an immunologist, I won't discuss those approaches here as they can be found in other publications.

Because my goal is to convince you of something that you may not see as obvious or even feasible, I have devoted several chapters in the beginning of the book to building the case for my central thesis. To start this process, chapter 1 is aimed at setting the stage by summarizing how research on cancer over the decades has had a significant positive impact on public health. Indeed, it is precisely because we have come so far that I refer to the cure for metastatic disease as the last mountaintop in cancer research.

What I will ultimately propose in this book is a new approach for treating end stage or metastatic cancer. Thus, it is important for readers who are not oncologists to have a basic understanding of how the traditional modes of cancer therapy work, and what their strengths and shortcomings are, and that is the subject of chapter 2.

As one progresses through this book it will become clear that a centerpiece of any novel strategy for metastatic cancer that does not involve chemotherapy or immunotherapy, will have to instead make better use of modern targeted cancer drugs. For that to make sense, one must have a basic understanding of the oncogenomic basis of cancer, and that is the subject of chapter 3. Cancer is, indeed, a genomic disease that is influenced by genetic factors and any strategy that will move us forward from where we are must use this fact as the starting point for better and more effective therapeutics.

As I mentioned above, we now have available to us massive amounts of genomic data from thousands of patients with cancer. In addition, we have amassed the same types of data from the hundreds of cancer cell lines that have been developed from biopsy tissues obtained from cancer patients. As I will argue throughout this book, the use of cell lines is absolutely necessary if we are going to put function to the otherwise descriptive genomic data that we have for patient-derived cancer tissues and cancer cells. Because of that necessity, chapter 4 is aimed at trying to convince the reader, and the skeptics, that cancer cell lines are excellent models of the specific disease that was experienced by the patients from which the cell lines were derived. There are some impressive and amazing organizations (The Broad Institute, the Wellcome Trust and others) that have invested millions of dollars to generate the kinds of functional genomics data that can only be obtained from cell lines, and we cannot ignore those data sets because of outmoded ideas about the usefulness of cancer cell lines. Thus, if you are one of those skeptics, you must read chapter 4. And even if you are one of the many thousands of cancer scientists around the world that use cancer cell lines in their work, you will also find some interesting tidbits in this chapter.

Chapter 5 is devoted to a description of how many groups and labs have used genome-scale essentiality screens in hundreds of cancer cell lines and how the data that has been obtained from these impressive experiments truly puts the <u>function</u> in functional genomics. The data derived from these kinds of experiments are what allows us to transform genomic data that are otherwise descriptive and noisy to data that are sharp and precise and, importantly, make predictions that are testable!

Thus, the first five chapters of this book are designed to set the stage for the data analysis sections that are presented in chapters 6 through 11. In these chapters I take a stepwise approach to the use of functional genomics for reverse engineering cancer cells. The first step is to use functional genomics to identify the genes that are most likely to be good targets of modern cancer drugs. Then, I examine how this approach can be used to determine, for those good genomic targets, the relationship between their essentialness and their sensitivity to drugs that target them. Next, I show how drug sensitivity data can be used as an alternative strategy to identify essential genes that are good drug targets.

The last three chapters of the book are aimed at tying this all together into what will be proposed as a novel strategy to reverse engineer metastatic cancer cells in patients. The ultimate strategy will include the application of Artificial Intelligence and Machine Learning methods to make predictions about drug sensitivity and resistance in individuals, and to leverage those predictions to design potent targeted drug combinations that can have high efficacy with little toxicity.

I wrap up the book with a reality check and a discussion of the paths that might be taken to implement the strategies ultimately developed as a result of this work so that effective clinical trials can be designed to provide the ultimate test of the methods and strategies that can come from developing reverse engineering strategies for metastatic cancer.

There is no cure for metastatic disease. Traditional methods involving chemotherapy alone have not worked. It is time for some alternative approaches.

ACKNOWLEDGEMENTS

In the nearly forty years that I have been working as a breast cancer researcher, I have had the opportunity and pleasure to work with many outstanding individuals. Among them are the many graduate students, medical students, post-doctoral fellows, and radiation oncology residents that have worked in my lab and whom I was proud to mentor. In addition, I've had the opportunity to work with and collaborate with some of the best cancer researchers in the world. It has been an honor for me to know and work with these fine scientists and clinicians. And over this span of forty years, I have published many papers with these individuals. The work presented in this monograph is my personal distillation of the topics and challenges that I consider to be most important and urgent in making future progress aimed at curing more patients with cancer. As such, there are data that are presented here that have not been published elsewhere, and I want to acknowledge the brilliant and talented people that were instrumental in generating the data shown in chapters 6 through 11.

I would first like to acknowledge Mr. Daniel Couch who brought his incredible skill and imagination to the generation of the MySQL database that underlies much of the work presented in these chapters. Daniel also wrote and launched all the data mining apps that are present on the SUM Breast Cancer Cell Line Knowledge Base (SLKBase). None of what has come later would have been possible without his work and talent.

Next, I'd like to acknowledge Mr. Kent Armeson. Kent is an outstanding biostatistician who wrote the R-scripts that resulted in the statistical analysis of the data shown as box and whisker plots and correlation plots shown in chapters 6 and 7.

I want to give a special acknowledgement to Dr. Steve Guest who worked with me for several years at the Karmanos Cancer Institute and the Medical University of South Carolina. Steve was the technical genius behind all of the genome-scale essentiality screens that we performed using the SUM breast cancer cell lines, among other cell lines. In addition, Steve worked with another brilliant computer scientist, Mr. Eric Czech, and together they performed the first-generation AI analysis of functional genomic data that resulted in a gene signature that can be used to predict sensitivity to the targeted drug Navitoclax. Some of the data from that analysis are shown in chapter 10.

And finally, I want to acknowledge Drs. Brittany Ivey and Jammie Mills, not only for the great work they did while in my lab at MUSC, but also for their critical reading of the manuscript.

The idea was fantastically, wildly improbable. But like most fantastically, wildly improbable ideas it was at least as worthy of consideration as a more mundane one to which the facts had been strenuously bent to fit. "

—Douglas Adams, "The Long Dark Tea-Time of the Soul"

CHAPTER 1

THE IMPACT OF 50 YEARS OF CANCER RESEARCH ON CANCER INCIDENCE, AND SURVIVAL

The goal of this book is to discuss what I consider to be the last mountaintop to be conquered on the war on cancer; how to effectively deal with clinically detectable metastatic disease. It should be obvious to everyone by now that despite our best efforts to improve the efficacy of local therapies for cancer, and for developing adjuvant chemotherapeutic approaches that make the emergence of clinical metastatic disease less likely, too many people still die of their cancer, and when they do, it is almost always because they succumb to their metastatic disease.

A brief primer on carcinogenesis and cancer prevention

Before we delve deeply into how we might use our understanding of cancer biology to conquer this last mountaintop of cancer research and clinical oncology, it is worthwhile to devote a bit of space at the outset to a discussion of how our understanding of the process of cancer development and carcinogenesis has had an enormous impact on cancer prevalence and cancer mortality. During the early years of the war on cancer, there were many aspects of cancer research that were not focused on how to best diagnose and treat cancer in patients. Rather, there were decades of work that were focused on understanding the basic biology of cancer development, and knowledge gained from this work was used to improve public health by identifying the causes of cancer in humans and instituting programs to reduce the cancer burden of the population.

Some of the biggest successes that led to the declining incidence of cancer were the result of a deep understanding of the process of cancer development in humans; a process known as carcinogenesis. When research in carcinogenesis began in the late 1960's we had almost no idea of the kinds of agents that cause cancer, and as a result, we were essentially ignorant of the mechanisms of human carcinogenesis.

However, significant progress in this field was made in the subsequent twenty or so years after the start of the war on cancer and the discoveries that were made resulted in a complex and essentially complete understanding of the molecular mechanisms by which chemical carcinogens, radiation carcinogens, and viral carcinogens cause cancer in humans (Poirier 2018; Penning 2011; Upton 1986). While the majority of this book will deal with advances in the treatment of cancer once it is diagnosed, the impact of our understanding of carcinogens and their mechanisms of action on the world-wide cancer burden cannot be overstated, because it is precisely because of our deep understanding of the molecular mechanisms of carcinogenesis that preventative measures at both personal and industrial levels were implemented that have had a large public health impact. For example, watch dial painters once used radioactive Radium to make the dials glow in the dark. As a result of our understanding of the mechanisms of radiation carcinogenesis, workers like these are no longer exposed to radioactive radium, and thus the bone cancers that occurred in those workers is no longer an industrial health issue. More recently, the understanding of the role of chemicals known as aromatic amines in the genesis of bladder and other cancers resulted in changes in the dye industry making this process safer for workers in this field and the prevention of many cancers. A particular type of aromatic amine called Aflatoxin, is the product of the mold *Aspergillus flavus* which for many years contaminated peanut crops, especially in African countries, and resulted in the development of liver cancer. There are many similar examples that involve many types of cancer-causing agents that are either no longer on the market, or are highly regulated, and thousands of papers have been published on this topic. Perhaps the most significant and far-reaching translation of the understanding of the mechanisms of chemical carcinogenesis to public health was the complete elucidation of how chemicals in cigarette smoke cause the development and progression of lung cancer in humans.

During the 1980s and much of the 1990's a mountain of circumstantial evidence accumulated that linked exposure to cigarette smoke, either primarily or secondarily, to the development of lung cancer in people. However, because a direct and causal mechanistic link between specific agents in cigarette smoke and lung cancer had not been definitely established, tobacco companies were able to argue that the evidence linking tobacco smoke to cancer and other diseases was only correlative and therefore, possibly not correct. Thus, they continued to argue that their products were safe or at least, might be safe.

All of that came to an end upon the definitive establishment of the specific types of mutations caused in specific genes known to be important in lung cancer, and the definitive demonstration that chemicals in cigarette smoke directly caused those mutations. Those final pieces of evidence at the molecular and genomic levels, the true smoking gun as it were, transformed what was once circumstantial and correlative evidence into a definitive link between smoking and lung cancer. And while this evidence was sufficient to counter all arguments from tobacco companies about the dangers of smoking, the more tangible and immediate impact came from the ability to use such data to file multiple class action lawsuits against tobacco companies that resulted in fines and settlements in the many billions of dollars. Some of that money was used to compensate victims of smoking related lung cancer, but some of that money, ironically, was also used to fund additional cancer research. As a result of all of this, the entire culture associated with cigarette smoking changed dramatically in the United States, and this has, no doubt, saved countless lives. All one has to do is remember the days when people actually smoked on elevators, in airplanes, and restaurants to realize the culture shift that resulted from a deep understanding of the molecular mechanisms of carcinogenesis (Hatsukami 2022).

One final anecdote that further illustrates the importance of basic research in carcinogenesis to cancer prevention is illustrated by the elucidation of the role of the Human Papilloma Virus type 16 (HPV-16) in the development of cervical cancer in woman and now, squamous cancers of the head and neck in women and men. There have been decades of research on the molecular mechanisms by which certain viruses cause cancer in animals, and there have been a few Nobel prizes awarded as a result. Even though several types of cancers in animals can be caused by different types of viruses, it turns out that a viral etiology of cancer in humans is quite rare. But one exception to that rule is the HPV-16 virus which is one of the causes of cervical cancer and squamous cancer of the head and neck. In this case, once again, the mechanistic evidence is clear, and we have a deep understanding of how two specific viral onco-proteins (the HPV-16 E6 and E7 proteins) cause these cancers. This definitive understanding has led to the development of vaccines against the HPV-16 virus that are now commonly administered to adolescent boys and girls. The wide-spread availability of HPV-16 vaccines will have a dramatic impact on the prevalence of these important cancer types, and this in turn, will result in dramatic reductions in morbidity and mortality from these types of cancers (David Jenkins 2019).

Thus, because of the progress that has been made in elucidating the mechanisms of carcinogenesis at the molecular and genomic levels, the burdens of cancer have been reduced dramatically. It is also clear that, given the nature of how cancer develops and progresses (to be discussed in more detail later), it is much better to prevent cancer than to try and cure it. Thus, research in carcinogenesis can be considered a major success in the war against cancer.

Key fundamental aspects of cancer biology. Over my career as a cancer researcher, I have given many lectures to medical students, medical residents, graduate students, and post-doctoral fellows (and the occasional intrepid undergrad) on what I refer to as the *fundamentals of cancer biology.* I always begin my lectures by making clear what I consider to be one of the most fundamental and poorly appreciated aspects of the biology of cancer; that is the apparent "latency" of these diseases in people. By latency, I mean the time that elapses between when the process of cancer development begins and when the disease can actually be diagnosed by some type of medical procedure or even the detection or palpation of a lump or tumor. Invariably, students in my class are surprised to learn that this latent period in humans for blood cancers such as leukemia and lymphoma is a decade or longer, and the latent period for the development of solid cancers such as lung cancer, breast cancer, colon cancers, etc. is on the order of 20 to 30 years! That means that by the time a clinician makes a definitive diagnosis of cancer in a patient, the development of that cancer has been ongoing for over 20 years. Thus, we should be careful with the term "early detection" because even the earliest of detections still occurs relatively late in the process of disease development. The importance of understanding this fundamental aspect of cancer biology to the ultimate goal of curing metastatic disease will become clearer later in this book.

The second fact that is related to the idea of cancer latency that my students are often surprised to learn but that is essential if one is to understand the biology of cancer is that cancer is a clonal disease. What that means is that the disease that is diagnosed as cancer in a patient had its origins in a single "transformed" cell. By the time the disease is diagnosed, the neoplasm as it is called, consists of tens of millions of cells all of which are the descendants of that single transformed cell. During the evolution of cancer many sub-clones develop that contribute to the emergence of a complex and heterogeneous neoplasm that play an important role in how the cancer responds to therapy. As the disease progresses the millions of cells present at diagnosis can grow to become over one billion cells, and once the disease progresses such that the tumor burden is on the order of one hundred billion cells, the patient will succumb to their disease. So that then, is the ultimate challenge of the Clinical Oncologist: first, how to detect cancer at its earliest stages when relatively fewer cancer cells are present, then how to eradicate as many of those few million cells as possible after the initial diagnosis, and then, how to prevent any residual cells from continuing to grow and proliferate to a point where the tumor burden becomes too great to be consistent with life. The process of cancer development from a single transformed cell to a few million cells at diagnosis, to billions of cells late in disease progression takes a long time, and a lot of biology happens during those years, all of which are important to the ultimate development of metastatic disease.

The stages of cancer progression. There have been many articles and books written on the biology of cancer progression and a detailed accounting of this process is beyond the scope of this book (for example see: (Coppola 2010)). However, before we delve into the main focus of the book, which is how to best leverage our understanding of cancer at the molecular level to develop 21st century treatment strategies ultimately aimed at curing metastatic disease, it's helpful at this point to say a few words about all of the biology that goes on during the so-called latent period between the time of the first transformed cell to the diagnosis of cancer. For many types of cancer, we can identify discreet stages of disease that occur before the cells of the neoplasm acquire full malignant potential. That statement on its own indicates that cancer in its earliest stages is not the life-threatening disease that it evolves to become. So then, what are some of the characteristics that the descendants of the first transformed cell acquire on their way to becoming fully malignant cells that can kill their host?

There are several, what we refer to as, hallmarks of cancer (Hanahan and Weinberg 2011). These hallmarks represent distinct biological features that cells acquire during their evolution to become cancer. For brevity's sake, I will list them here, but keep in mind, that during the process of cancer evolution, cells can acquire these features in any order, though one of them in particular (genomic instability) is important for the acquisition of the others and for the emergence of sub-clones within the neoplasm.

- Cellular immortality. Yes, cancer cells, unlike your normal cells can live forever.
- Independence of proliferative signals from hormones or growth factors

- Resistance to growth inhibitory signals
- Resistance to signals that would induce programmed cell death
- Ability to evade immune surveillance
- Acquisition of genomic instability
- Acquisition of cellular motility
- Acquisition of ability to invade surrounding normal healthy tissue
- Ability to enter and exit the vasculature and proliferate in new sites

Early in the evolution of a malignant neoplasm, cells might exhibit only a few of these hallmarks and this is one of the reasons why early detection can be so important, because once cells acquire all of these hallmarks and become fully malignant and metastatic, clinical treatment becomes more difficult and sometimes impossible. And, as I indicated above, the acquisition of these properties takes time and occurs in discreet steps that are the result of specific alterations in the genome of the cancer cells.

Now, with that as a background, let's now begin a consideration of how understanding cancer biology plays a role in cancer therapy, both traditionally and in the future.

CHAPTER 2

THE THREE ARMS OF TRADITIONAL CLINICAL ONCOLOGY

Now that we have a better understanding of what patients and oncologists are dealing with once the diagnosis of cancer is made, I will provide a brief overview of the strategies that are used to combat the disease. Before that though, we need to introduce one more fundamental aspect of the biology of human cancer, and that has to do with what we refer to as cancer progression.

We have established that cancer originates in a single cell in a single tissue and is the result of many rounds of cell division that takes place over decades. That single transformed cell ultimately gives rise to a tumor or a lump that can be detected directly or by some of our newest imaging techniques (X-rays, ultrasounds, CT scans, MRI scans, etc.) The lump or tumor that is detected is referred to as the *primary tumor* or as *local disease* because it is diagnosed in the same tissue that was the home of the original transformed cell. Thus, a single transformed cell in one of the milk ducts of breast tissue can give rise to a tumor that is detected in the breast. The same is true for transformed cells in lung tissue giving rise to a lung tumor and transformed cells in the colon giving rise to a colon polyp and then a colon cancer. So, once again, the primary tumor is what is referred to as local disease. If local disease is all we had to deal with, cancer would not be the clinical problem that it is. Indeed, a benign tumor is one that develops locally and remains in the local region throughout its natural history because the cells of a benign neoplasm do not have the capacity to invade normal tissue or the vasculature. As a result, it is rare for anyone to die of benign disease. The opposite of benign disease is malignant disease, and this is what we are referring to when we use the term cancer. The fundamental difference between benign and malignant disease is that malignant cancer cells acquire the ability to become motile and invasive. That is, the cells don't just stay put within the tumor they have formed, but rather, the cells burrow away from the primary tumor invading and destroying the normal cells along the way. And as part of that process, these malignant cancer cells worm their way into the vasculature; the small blood vessels and lymphatic vessels that are, no pun intended, the lifeblood of every living tissue. Once these malignant cancer cells gain access to the vasculature, the cells can be rapidly distributed throughout the body. Then, sometimes the cells worm their way back out of the circulation and into a tissue far distant from the primary tumor. This dissemination of cancer cells and the establishment of secondary tumors at sites far distant from the primary tumor is the process of metastasis. As I have already mentioned and will be discussed in great detail later, dealing with metastatic cancer is the ultimate challenge in clinical oncology. Thus, finding novel ways to cure metastatic disease is, therefore, the last mountaintop in clinical oncology and it is a challenge that remains to be conquered.

Given our general understanding of the progression of human cancer, let's return to the goals of the three arms of Oncology which are: surgical oncology, radiation oncology, and medical oncology.

Surgical Oncology. As we discussed above, a primary tumor that is detected either by the patient or their doctor usually consists of from 1 million cells to about 10 million cells and sometimes more depending on the size of the primary tumor. In Clinical Oncology it is well known that size does indeed matter. The smaller the tumor that is first detected and treated the better the outcome of the patient, and this makes sense in terms of how cancer progresses. So, the first line of attack in the clinical battle against cancer almost always involves a surgical oncologist whose goal is to remove as many of those cancer cells as possible using the most modern methods of surgical oncology. As a friend and former colleague of mine used to say, 'a chance to cut is a chance to cure'. He is obviously a surgeon.

Keep in mind that when the surgeon removes a primary tumor, he or she can see the lump itself and they can see what they consider to be the margins of that lump, but they can't see the cancer cells themselves. Thus, the goal of any surgical procedure for cancer is to remove the entire primary tumor and obtain "clear margins", i.e., edges free of cancer cells. It is the job of the surgical pathologist to examine the tumor once it's removed and determine if indeed the margins are clear of cancer cells. This is critical because once again, it is well known that if the surgeon truly "gets it all" the patient is cured of their disease. Full stop. And it follows then that the smaller the tumor is, the more likely it is that the surgical procedure removes every last cancer cell from a patient's body.

As a result of decades of clinical research, we have a very good understanding of the outcomes that can be expected for many types of cancer following a surgical intervention. And we know that in some cases, particularly those in which the primary tumor is large or for which the surgery is difficult and complex, e.g., the Whipple procedure for pancreas cancer, if nothing else is done beyond the surgery, some patients will recure with the same cancer at the primary site either months or years later, and this is never a good outcome. Indeed, these so-called local recurrences can occur even in patients who had clear margins after the primary surgery, although this is less common.

Radiation Oncology. Enter the radiation oncologist. The field of radiation oncology is highly complex and makes use of cutting-edge technology in terms of radiation beam energy and design, and real-time imaging of the tumor being treated. Although in some case, radiation treatment is the primary modality for the treatment of primary cancers, for the purposes of this discussion, I want to focus on the role of the radiation oncologist as a partner to the surgical oncologist in achieving so-called "local control" of a primary tumor. Although there are now many examples of how this clinical partnership has had a great impact on cure rates for cancer, the specific example of how these modalities are used to treat breast cancer is illustrative of the broader field.

It wasn't very long ago that the standard surgical procedure for a woman (or a man) diagnosed with breast cancer was the modified radical mastectomy; a procedure where the entire breast was removed along with regional lymph nodes. This was, indeed, a radical strategy aimed at ensuring that the entire primary tumor was removed from the patient. As a result, local recurrence rates following this procedure were quite low. Over the years, the field of surgical oncology has moved toward the use of less radical and more conservative procedures and for breast cancer, the current standard of care is to perform a lumpectomy instead of a modified radical mastectomy, whenever possible. This procedure, which strives to remove only the tumor and leave as much of the breast intact as possible, yields a better cosmetic result and has been a factor in women being more amenable to early detection strategies like mammography. However, clinical research in this area demonstrated quite convincingly that, in terms of local control, i.e., the rate of local recurrence after surgery, lumpectomy was not as effective as the modified radical mastectomy. Local recurrence rates following lumpectomy alone were unacceptably high, which puts patients at higher risk of distant metastasis later in life. So, as I indicated above, this is where the radiation oncologist enters the picture.

The finding of unacceptably high local recurrence rates following lumpectomy alone meant that, despite best efforts to obtain clear margins, some residual cancer cells are left behind. Over time, these cells can grow into a new tumor at the primary site. In an attempt to combat this and retain lumpectomy as a primary strategy, studies were conducted to determine if administration of local radiation at the primary site after lumpectomy could reduce rates of local recurrence. The idea is that, following surgery with a course of radiation will kill any residual cancer cells left behind by the surgeon, and thus reduce or eliminate local recurrence. The clinical studies that examined the efficacy of lumpectomy followed by radiation were highly successful, and we now know that lumpectomy plus radiation is just as effective at achieving local control of breast cancer as modified radical mastectomy. This was a major advance in the treatment of breast cancer, which is the second most common cancer in women (Speers and Pierce 2016).

In an interesting twist on the success of this dual modality treatment, it was found that for some patients, the size of the primary breast cancer is too large to make lumpectomy feasible. For these patients, radiation therapy is sometimes given first to shrink the tumor and make it amenable to lumpectomy instead of the more radical surgery.

Over the years, there has been an increasing trend for more and more conservative surgeries for many types of cancer and in these cases, the combination of conservative surgery plus radiation therapy has served to optimize local control rates and minimize the rates of local recurrence. This is a great success story in clinical oncology.

Why then, do these state-of-the-art methods for eradicating the primary cancer not result in more cures of disease? The reason for this is because for those patients that don't recur at the site of the primary tumor, they can recur at distant sites, because as we discussed earlier, malignant cancer cells have that ability to invade the vasculature and travel to distant sites in the body. So, when a patient is treated locally with surgery plus radiation and recurs months or years later at one or more *distant* sites, that means that *at the time of surgery*, some of those cancer cells had *already moved away* from the primary tumor and were lurking undetected in other tissues of the body. Keep in mind, that all patients that are treated to achieve local control also undergo extensive imaging and screening to search for the presence of secondary tumors at distant sites. Most often, the results of these tests are negative. This means that from a clinical perspective, patients who complete their local therapy and have been screened for distant disease are considered to be "clinically disease free". However, we know that some of these patients are not completely disease free because some fraction of them will recur at distant sites months or years later (as late as 15 years in some cases!).

Recall our discussion on the diagnosis of primary cancers. We said that primary tumors, when detected, usually consist of one-million cancer cells or more. Why can't we detect cancer at earlier stages, i.e., when there are fewer cancer cells? For starters, such a small tumor doesn't usually cause any symptoms, so patients don't know they have them. Secondly, our detection methods are not sensitive enough to know when a patient has only a few hundred or a few thousand cancer cells in their body. So, when patients who are considered to be clinically disease free after their primary cancer treatment recur at distant sites later, it's because there were a small number of cancer cells lurking at one or more of these distant sites, and they too went undetected until they grew into tumors of a detectable size, or when they caused symptoms. Such patients are said to have had "occult metastatic disease".

In situations like this, we can't determine which specific patients have occult metastatic disease, but we do have a good idea of the *likelihood* that a patient has such occult disease. Knowing the odds that a patient who is clinically disease free actually has occult metastatic disease can be used to make a determination of the potential for benefit of chemotherapy following the treatment of the primary tumor.

Medical Oncology. Enter the Medical Oncologist. The primary goal of the medical oncologist is to attack, what we refer to as, systemic disease. Systemic disease is the opposite of local disease. Systemic disease is the result of the process of metastasis in which the entire body *system* is at risk for the emergence of metastatic cancer. The tool used by medical oncologists to treat systemic disease is primarily chemotherapy.

Over the decades, medicinal chemists, pharmaceutical companies, and medical oncologists have developed a dizzying array of chemotherapeutic drugs. Often these drugs are used in combinations that have been painstakingly tested in clinical trials before being administered to patients. For the purposes of this discussion, it's important that people understand that most chemotherapeutic drugs are blunt instruments. That is, they are designed primarily to kill proliferating cells and not necessarily cancer cells. Since one of the defining characteristics of cancer cells is their propensity to undergo cell division (proliferation) in an uncoordinated and unregulated manner, chemotherapeutic drugs are excellent at killing cancer cells. The problem is that cancer cells are not the only cells in the body that are proliferating. For example, the bone marrow is full of rapidly dividing cells whose job it is to consistently replenish the supply of red and white blood cells found in the circulation. Similarly, there are millions of proliferating cells lining the intestines whose job it is to continuously replenish the cells that are vital to the maintenance of the gastro-intestinal track, and to be sure that nutrients and water are absorbed from foods to be used as the energy that fuels life. The skin is another organ that is constantly turning over (hence house dust!) and thus the basal later (bottom) of the epidermis consists of rapidly proliferating cells.

As I mentioned above, chemotherapeutic drugs are blunt instruments and that means that these drugs are effective at killing all proliferating cells, not just cancer cells. It is this non-specificity that is the basis for the common side effects that are associated with chemotherapy; hair loss; nausea, vomiting and diarrhea, and various types of anemia. Thus, the medical oncologist is always trying to use chemotherapeutic drugs to kill as many cancer cells as possible without killing the patient with the drugs. Indeed, a large part of the training of medical oncologists revolves around the medical practices used to treat the toxicities that are caused by the chemotherapeutic drugs, and there have been great advances in these treatments. In the cases where there are a relatively few metastatic cancer cells in the body, chemotherapy can effectively kill essentially all the cancer cells without doing too much harm to the patient. In these cases, chemotherapy is curative. We know this because measurements of the overall survival rates in groups of patients who receive this type of chemotherapy are better than for those that don't. More often than not though, chemotherapy reduces tumor burden without eradicating all of the cancer cells and in these cases, the patients recur at distant sites months or years after their chemotherapy. Often, patients will recur later than they would have, had they not received chemotherapy, and thus, the chemotherapy can add years of life for the patient. But such patients are not cured.

Given that recurrence is possible following chemotherapy, I want to get back to the course of cancer treatment that was discussed above and now highlight the role of the medical oncologist in affecting cures for patients. Above, I described a scenario where a patient was treated with surgery and radiation to achieve local control of the cancer, and in which screening for overt metastatic disease indicated that the patient was clinically disease free. Now, imagine that this is a situation in which the medical oncologist knows, based on years of clinical trial data for patients with similar characteristics of the primary tumor, that the patient has a 25% chance of having occult metastatic disease, even though it is not presently detectable. What does the medical oncologist and the patient do with this information?

In modern medical oncology, when these situations exist, and they are common, the standard of care is often to treat *all* the patients with a chemotherapeutic regimen that is considered “well tolerated” by most patients. This type of treatment is referred to as *adjuvant* (meaning added or additional) chemotherapy. One can see right away the advantages and disadvantages of this approach. The advantage is that by treating patients who have a relatively small number of cancer cells lurking somewhere in the body, the chances of killing all those remaining cancer cells without undue harm to the patient are relatively high. And indeed, adjuvant chemotherapy has contributed to improved *cure* rates for many types of cancer. The disadvantage of this strategy is that, in this scenario, 75% of the patients with similar types of disease will receive chemotherapy even though they don’t have *any* occult metastatic cells lurking in their bodies. Thus, these patients were actually cured by their local therapy, but there was no definitive way to know this. Thus, they receive no benefit from the chemotherapy, but they will incur all the side effects. For the majority of patients who receive a cancer diagnosis, this is a gamble they are willing to take. As a result, this type of adjuvant chemotherapy has become the standard of care for many types of cancer because the consequences of recurring with full blown metastatic disease are so dire.

One of the most exciting areas of research in medical oncology today has the goal of developing more sophisticated ways to identify the specific patients that are most likely to have occult metastatic disease, and which are therefore most likely to benefit from the chemotherapy. There are already some excellent examples of strategies that are being used effectively to spare patients from chemotherapy who don’t require it (Curtit et al. 2017; Markopoulos 2013; Carlson and Roth 2013). Increasingly, clinicians are making use of genome sequencing methods to examine circulating DNA in the blood of cancer patients, as detecting genomic alterations present in the cancer cells in the blood can be an early sign of the presence of occult metastatic cells. There are also new genomic strategies that make predictions about the likelihood of recurrence based on the genomic features present in the primary cancer. These genomic signatures are being used today to spare many patients from chemotherapy that they don’t require.

There is no cure for metastatic disease

Earlier we used breast cancer treatment as an example of how surgery and radiation therapy have been used to virtually eliminate local recurrences of breast cancer. And yet, even though most women who are diagnosed with breast cancer do not die of their disease, too many women still do. Why? The reason is that when breast cancer cells disseminate throughout the body they go to places like the bone, the liver, and the brain. And in so doing, these metastatic cells can develop into dozens to hundreds of individual metastatic nodules. As these *secondary* tumors grow, they destroy the normal cells that are present in that secondary site. The liver is a remarkable organ, and we can live with only about half of our liver. Thus, breast cancer cells metastatic to liver can grow for a long time before they cause symptoms associated with liver disease. When these cancer cells destroy the function of more than half of the liver, the patient will die. The same is true for loss of function of brain tissue and bone marrow. In fact, it is the proliferation of metastatic breast cancer cells in bone that is the cause of so much pain endured by breast cancer patients once these metastases are established in bone and bone marrow.

So now you see the problem. Because once patients present with *clinically detectable* metastatic cancer, they are essentially *not curable*. The term, 'there is no cure for metastatic disease' is *almost* as true today as it was 30 years ago. And thus, this is where we need to do much better and develop novel strategies to get us to the top of this last mountaintop.

Before we delve further into what I consider to be potentially viable strategies that can get us to this mountaintop, it's instructive to discuss how medical oncologists use chemotherapy to combat clinically detectable metastatic cancer currently because as we will see, these methods can be effective, but they also can contribute to the problem that we are trying to deal with, and sometimes make it worse.

Chemotherapy for overt metastatic disease

There are now several different types of imaging strategies that can be used by oncologists to not only detect the presence of secondary cancers at metastatic sites, but also accurately measure their size, their metabolic activity, and their growth rates. Thus, when oncologists use chemotherapy to treat patients with overt metastatic disease, they use these imaging methods to determine just how well or poorly the drugs being used are working. For the most common types of cancer, there are standard chemotherapeutic regimens used to treat patients with metastatic disease, and indeed, as a result of a number of clinical trials, there are often first line, second line, and even third line standard approaches for systemic therapy. In other cases, for example in ovarian cancer, while there is a clear standard of chemotherapy treatment that follows surgical removal of the tumor mass, there are no clearly defined second or third line chemotherapy regimens for this type of cancer. As a result, the choice of chemotherapy that is used to treat recurrent ovarian cancer is left to the discretion and experience of the oncologist, in consultation with the patient.

As may be obvious by now, the reason that there is a need for multiple lines of chemotherapeutic strategies is because when patients develop overt metastatic disease and are treated with chemotherapy, the most commonly observed scenario is for patients to have a good response to the therapy initially with sometimes dramatic reductions in tumor burden. However, the durability of these remissions is variable. One thing is almost certain; a patient will eventually recur and require further treatment. Depending on the aggressiveness of the disease, remissions of metastatic lesions can last for months or even years, and sometimes lesions in some metastatic sites respond better than those in other sites in the same individual. Thus, these chemotherapeutic strategies have significant benefit to the patient as they can add years of life for the patient and their family. However, at some point, the patient will recur with lesions in the same metastatic sites or even different sites. At that point, the medical oncologist generally starts the patient on a different cocktail of chemotherapeutic drugs and the process begins again. A typical scenario is that as patients proceed through multiple lines of chemotherapy, the duration of the remissions becomes shorter and ultimately, the patient fails to respond significantly to the drugs. These lack of responses are compounded by the accumulation of the toxic side effects of the multiple chemotherapy drugs, and a most visible result of this in patients is a clear acceleration of the aging process. Taking chemotherapy for cancer is not for the faint of heart.

As a result of the process that I just described, while chemotherapy for metastatic disease does provide significant and tangible benefit to the patient, the patients are rarely if ever cured of their disease. So, why is that?

There are two important limiting factors to the efficacy of chemotherapy for patients with measurable metastatic disease. First, there is the well-known and understood phenomenon of acquired drug resistance and this ultimately limits the usefulness of any chemotherapeutic drug (Pastan and Gottesman 1987; Periti and Mini 1989; Dickson and Gottesman 1990). As a result, while the responses to the chemotherapy may be excellent during the early phases of therapy, the effectiveness of the drugs begins to lessen over time, and this necessitates changing to other drugs. Unfortunately, there is something known as multi-drug resistance which results in patients becoming resistant to not only the first drugs that were used, but many other chemotherapeutic drugs as well, even though the patient has never experienced those drugs.

The second issue, which in some ways is related to the first, is that the drugs themselves are genotoxic, i.e., they induce changes in the DNA of the cancer cells that are not killed by the treatment. Because most drugs used in chemotherapy attack the DNA of cancer cells directly or indirectly as part of their mechanism of action, some of the cells that survive the toxic effects of the drugs acquire new mutations or genomic alterations, and the metastatic lesions that recur are different at the genomic level from the lesions that were originally treated. This effect serves to compound the problem of acquired drug resistance. Together, these two phenomena ultimately limit the long-term effectiveness of chemotherapy in patients with metastatic disease, and this is the reason why, even today, patients with metastatic disease are rarely cured using chemotherapy alone.

So now, we see the problem clearly. As a result of decades of research both in the laboratory and the clinic, we understand some of the best ways to prevent cancer, we understand how to control cancer at the local or primary site, and we have made strides using adjuvant chemotherapy to prevent the recurrence of overt metastatic disease for patients with occult metastatic disease. But, despite all of that progress, once patients progress and show signs of overt, clinically detectable metastasis, the ultimate prognosis is grim. And thus, the treatment and cure of metastatic disease does, as I have said, represent the ultimate challenge and the last mountaintop to be conquered in the war on cancer.

If, as I have pointed out here, we have done all that we can in our attempts to cure metastatic disease using traditional chemotherapeutic drugs, what other approaches might we develop to ultimately get us to the top of this mountain? There are two emerging strategies that offer hope for the ultimate cure of metastatic cancer: immunotherapy, and therapy using the newest generation of targeted cancer drugs. In the pages that follow, I will not spend significant time discussing immunotherapy, as there are other excellent sources of information on these newly emerging and sometimes highly effective modalities. Rather, the main goal of this book is to discuss what I believe are the reasons why targeted cancer therapies can lead to great breakthroughs in this area, and the work that needs to be done to make further progress in this area. And as you will see, there is much to be done.

CHAPTER 3

THE ONCOGENOMIC BASIS OF CANCER

I have now introduced the term "targeted cancer drugs" and have offered some hope that these new types of cancer drugs can be the pathway that leads us to the mountaintop. So, what are these so-called targeted cancer drugs and how do they differ from traditional chemotherapeutic drugs?

As I discussed earlier, traditional chemotherapeutic drugs are blunt instruments that are designed to kill virtually any type of proliferating or dividing cells. Using traditional chemotherapeutic drugs to kill cancer cells is sort of like trying to fix a Swiss watch with a sledgehammer; you can ultimately cause as much harm as good. So, if traditional chemo drugs are blunt instruments, targeted cancer drugs are, as the term implies, designed to be precision instruments that have direct and profound effects on cancer cells while having little or no effect on normal cells. To understand how such drugs came to exist and why some of them have already found their place in standard cancer therapy, it is important that we understand more about the genomic basis of cancer development. It is because of the research that elucidated the genomic basis of cancer that targeted cancer drugs came into existence in the first place.

Whenever I teach cancer biology to clinicians and researchers, I always take time at the outset to define clearly what I mean by the term "genomics" and how that differs from the term "genetics". This is important because as we will see, cancer is a genomic disease that is influenced by genetic factors.

Both genomics and genetics have to do with the DNA that is present in almost every living cell. DNA is what genes are made which, directly or indirectly, control just about everything a living cell does. The difference between genomics and genetics is that genomics refers to the state of the DNA in all cells of the body *except* the so-called germ-line cells, i.e., the sperm cells in men and the egg cells in women. As a result, any changes that occur in the DNA of most cells of the body, while possibly affecting the disease state of the tissue in which those cells reside, can never be passed on to offspring. By contrast, changes or mutations in DNA that occur in the germ line cells can and often are passed on to offspring. Characteristics of the genome that are heritable therefore defines genetics and distinguishes it from genomics. And, as I indicated above, cancer is both a genomic and a genetic disease.

Let's spend more time discussing the genomics of cancer. We have known for decades that the process of cancer development starts with carcinogen-induced damage to the DNA of the cells that become transformed into the precursors of cancer. Earlier, I discussed how research in human carcinogenesis resulted in a deep understanding of the kinds of agents that cause cancer, and at the molecular level, how that all happens. The upshot from all this work is that we came to understand that the agents that cause cancer have specific chemical properties that allow them to not only damage DNA, but cause mutations in the DNA code that can alter the properties of the gene that has acquired the mutation. This, in turn, can alter the behavior of the cells with the mutation. It is the ability of carcinogens to cause mutations in DNA that is the basis for the "transformation" of normal cells into the precursors of cancer.

If cancer causing agents initiate the process of cancer development and progression by causing mutations in DNA, are there specific genes in the human genome that are at risk for such changes, or can cancer be caused by damage to virtually any gene in the genome? As a result of the heroic work of the scientific community that led to the elucidation of the entire human genome sequence, we know that the human genome consists of roughly 20,000 different genes that are spread across our 23 chromosomes (Guyer and Collins 1993; Collins 1997; Fink and Collins 1997). All human cells (except for those germ line cells) have 46 chromosomes because there are two copies of each chromosome (one from mom and one from dad), thus we have two copies of all our genes. So again, do all 20,000 genes play a role in cancer? No.

It is beyond the scope of this book to describe how research on cancer led us to understand the sub-set of genes in the human genome that play a direct role in cancer development when they are damaged because of exposure to carcinogens. Suffice it to say that we know of about 500 of the 20,000 genes that play a role in cancer, and most cancers are the result of DNA alterations in an even smaller subset of genes: perhaps as few as 50 to 100. But given that our understanding of cancer genomics has allowed us to focus our efforts on a pretty small section of the genome, progress in our understanding the molecular basis of cancer has proceeded with lightning speed.

Allow me now to take a moment to define a couple of terms. The set of 500 or so genes that we know can play a role in driving the process of cancer development are referred to as "proto-oncogenes". We use the term *proto* to indicate that when these genes are normal and have not been damaged by carcinogens, they play important regulatory roles in the biology of our normal cells. Indeed, these genes are essential to life. But, when these proto-oncogenes acquire specific types of DNA damage that can transform a cell, these proto-oncogenes become *activated* and are then referred to as *oncogenes*. If I'm doing a good job explaining this, you may be starting to see where this is going with respect to targeted cancer drugs. Yes?

Okay, is the damage caused in the DNA of proto-oncogenes that causes them to become activated oncogenes random or specific? As it happens, activation is the result of highly specific, and thus rare types of DNA damage. This is one of the reasons why everyone doesn't have cancer all the time! Essentially, there are three types of DNA damage that can activate proto-oncogenes into oncogenes: gene amplification, point mutation, or gene-rearrangement. Let's take these one at a time.

As I indicated above, all our cells have two copies of every gene in the genome: one from mom and one from dad. Two copies is normal. Sometimes during the process of cancer development, the genome can become destabilized resulting in gene-amplification events that lead to the acquisition of extra copies of certain genes. That is, some parts of some chromosomes replicate themselves incorrectly resulting in small regions of the genome that are amplified, which results in a small number of genes having more, and sometimes a lot more, than two copies. These gene amplification events are the driving force behind the development of many types of solid human cancers, such as breast cancer, colon cancer, and others (Beroukhim et al. 2010; Santarius et al. 2010). Now, if an amplification event in a certain genomic region results in a growth advantage of that cell over the normal and neighboring cells, then those cells can expand and form the early stages of a neoplasm. More on this below.

The second type of DNA damage that can be "transforming" is the acquisition of specific point mutations within a gene. For this to make sense, we need to have a basic understanding of what we mean by the term 'mutation'. Every gene in the genome is essentially a code, that is, it is an instruction that tells the cell how to make a specific protein. Thus, the one gene-one-protein hypothesis has been part of the central dogma of biology for over a century. So then, the DNA sequence of a gene is a specific instruction of how to make a specific protein. The DNA code is made up of a string (a long string!) of so-called bases, which are adenine, thymine, guanine, and cytosine. Hence forth, we will simply refer to these bases by their first initial: A, T, C, and G. Here is what a DNA code for a small piece of a gene might look like:

A-T-G-A-A-T-T-A-C-A-G-T-C-A-C (imagine this thousands of bases long and you are starting to get the idea of what one gene "looks" like).

But wait, the DNA code is not just a linear sequence because it is organized into groups of three bases, which are known as codons. So, as far as the cell is concerned, the sequence shown above actually "reads" like this:

A-T-G A-A-T T-A-C A-G-T C-A-C

As pointed out above, a gene codes for a protein and a protein is a long chain of molecules called amino acids. There are 22 different amino acids that can be used in an almost infinite number of combinations to make the tens of thousands of proteins present in your cells. So, the code shown above is read by the cell as an instruction to link the following five amino acids together:

Methionine, Asparagine, Tyrosine, Serine and Histidine (MET-ASN-TYR-SER-HIS)

So now, imagine that there has been a mutation that occurred in the third codon shown above that changed the sequence from T-A-C to T-G-C. In this case, the amino acid in the third position would change from a Tyrosine (TYR) to a Cysteine (CYS). Now, given that it is the precise amino acid sequence of a protein that gives it it's function, changing even one critical amino acid can have a profound effect on the biological activity of that protein. Now, imagine that there was a mutation that changed the T-A-C to T-A-G. The T-A-G codon is actually the signal to the cell to terminate the synthesis of the protein. So, were this to happen, the cell would try to make a protein that was missing the last two amino acids. Such a protein would certainly have a different biology activity than the normal version.

In case you're wondering how the cell transcribes the information from the DNA code, which is found in the cell's nucleus, to the part of the cell outside of the nucleus that is responsible for building proteins, the molecules that do this are called messenger RNAs. As a result of our recent pandemic and the novel vaccines that resulted, virtually everyone on the planet has now heard of messenger RNA, and this may also give you some added insight as to how these vaccines work, but we digress.

Back to our story of how point mutations in proto-oncogenes can activate them into transforming oncogenes. If a specific point mutation changes the amino acid in the protein coded for by the oncogene in a way that basically hyperactivates the function of that protein, that can be the transforming event that plays a critical role in the process of cancer development (Sekiya T et al. 1985; Bargmann, Hung, and Weinberg 1986; Cohen and Levinson 1988; Roussel et al. 1988). This is exactly the mechanism by which point mutations can "activate" proto-oncogenes to oncogenes during the process of cancer development. And, because mutation events that can activate proto-oncogenes to oncogenes are very precise and hence very rare, there are relatively few known and recurrent point mutations in known oncogenes. This makes identifying them much easier.

There is another side to the mutation story that must be discussed here, even though it doesn't directly have to do with the activation of oncogenes. In cancer biology, there are a set of genes that act as counterpoints to oncogenes. These genes are called tumor suppressor genes and, as the name suggests, their role is to keep cells from becoming cancer cells (Marshall 1991; Weinberg 1991). Thus, during cancer progression, not only are oncogenes (the gas) activated, but tumor suppressor genes (the brakes) are inactivated. Some of you may already know that most mutations that occur in genes are deleterious and as a result damage the gene's function rather than activating it or enhancing it. That's because it's a lot easier to break a gene than to cause it to become hyper-active. Thus, most point mutations that occur in cancer do so in tumor suppressor genes and that is how their function is lost during cancer progression.

Okay, back to the oncogene story. The third basic mechanism of oncogene activation is a process called gene re-arrangement. Imagine that breaks occur in two chromosomes in a way that results in a piece of one chromosome being connected to a broken piece of a different chromosome. This process is referred to as a reciprocal translocation and it happens more often in cancer then you might think (Cory 1986; Haluska and Croce 1987; Haluska, Tsujimoto, and Croce 1987; Groffen and Heisterkamp 1989; Rowley 1990). This process can generate some interesting forms of activated oncogenes. The most famous such activating event occurs in a type of leukemia called chronic myelogenous leukemia (CML) (Rowley 1990). In this disease, a piece of chromosome 9 breaks off and gets reconnected to a piece of chromosome 22. In so doing, a piece of one gene that was on chromosome 9 becomes fused with a piece of the gene on chromosome 22. The result of this process is a new gene, a so-called fusion gene. In CML the gene from chromosome 9 is called BCR and the gene on chromosome 22 is called ABL. Interestingly, while the normal form of the ABL gene codes for a protein whose function is precisely regulated by the cell, the BCR-ABL fusion protein is basically stuck in the on position, and is therefore completely unregulated and thus, activated. And we know from years of research on this disease that this reciprocal translocation is an activating event for the ABL oncogene. This is one example of how specific gene rearrangement events can result in activation of oncogenes. There are many others that result in activation of other oncogenes as this is a common mode of oncogene activation in leukemias.

By now, you might be wondering why I'm telling you all of this as this may be more biology than you bargained for when you picked up this book. The answer to your question has to do with one of the most fundamental and important aspects of cancer biology, the theory of Oncogene Addiction.

The term Oncogene Addiction was proposed by the late Dr. Bernard Weinstein of Columbia University (B. Weinstein 1987; I.B. Weinstein et al. 1997; I.B. Weinstein and Joe 2006; I.B. Weinstein and Joe 2008). As it was proposed by Dr. Weinstein, "cancer cells contain multiple genetic and epigenetic abnormalities. Despite this complexity, their growth and survival can often be impaired by the inactivation of a single oncogene." Thus, cancer cells become addicted to their oncogenes such that, any disruption in the function of those genes leads to the death of the cancer cells. And as you may have figured out by now, the theory of oncogene addiction is the basis for the development of many targeted cancer drugs, as these drugs are specifically designed to attack and inactivate the driving oncogenes in cancer cells.

Oncogene Addiction in Patients. Over many years of cancer research, a large volume of experimental data has been generated in model systems of cancer that supported the theory of oncogene addiction in many types of human cancer. And yet, no matter how likely it appears that a theory is correct, definitive proof can only be obtained when the experimental results are translated to results in patients with cancer.

In the case of the BCR-ABL fusion oncogene discussed above, the experimental evidence was so powerful, that Dr. Brian Drucker and colleagues set out to develop a drug that could block the activity of the altered version of the ABL protein in CML cells (B. Druker et al. 1996; B. Druker, Talpaz, et al. 2001; B.J. Druker, Sawyers, et al. 2001; Deininger and Druker 2003; B.J. Druker 2008). Without going in to too much detail, the protein coded for by the ABL proto-oncogene is an enzyme (specifically a tyrosine kinase), meaning that its role in life is to catalyze specific chemical reactions in cells with efficiency and accuracy. For aficionados who want to know more, ABL like many oncogenes, are specific types of enzymes called kinases, and you can google more about that if you'd like. From a drug development perspective, there are many advantages to designing drugs that block the action of enzymes. One of the things I didn't tell you about proteins earlier is that, not only are they made up of a long chain of amino acids arranged in a specific order. Because of that order, the protein molecules fold, like origami, into highly precise three-dimensional structures. The shapes of these molecules are key to their enzymatic activities. Such enzyme molecules often have grooves that are designed to fit with other molecules that are part of the chemical reaction that they catalyze. So, in making a drug that blocks the activity of an enzyme, one needs to identify or synthesize a molecule that fits into that groove, thus blocking it from interacting with the proper molecule. Thus, an enzyme is like a lock with a groove that fits the key in a precise way and a drug is like a key that fits in the groove but won't open the lock. If the actual key can't get into the groove, the door won't unlock. Obviously, this isn't as easy as it sounds, but over the years, medicinal chemists have become very good at designing molecules that are excellent inhibitors of the activity of enzymes by blocking these enzymatic grooves or pockets.

Of the many candidate inhibitors that were designed to block the activity of the BCR-ABL oncogene activity in CML, the one that worked best in experimental studies, was called imatinib (B. Druker et al. 1996; B. Druker, Talpaz, et al. 2001). Because imatinib was so effective blocking the growth and survival of CML cells with the BCR-ABL oncogene, but not cells with the normal ABL gene/protein, this candidate drug was eventually tested in clinical trials on patients with CML. There are many excellent sources that readers can consult to learn more about the specifics of these clinical trials, but for our purposes here, let me summarize by saying that the trials were highly successful, and imatinib, which is now known as Gleevec, became standard therapy for patients diagnosed with CML. Indeed, this drug is so potent against CML that, for patients who are diagnosed early in their clinical course, when the BCR-ABL gene is the sole driver of the disease, imatinib can cure patients with high efficiency (Deininger and Druker 2003). Thus, this drug completely changed how CML is treated clinically and has had a profound impact on the survival of patients with this type of leukemia. Thus, in this case, the theory of oncogene addiction was correct.

There is a second success story that helped to further the optimism behind the theory of oncogene addiction and the development of targeted drugs for cancer. This second success came following the identification of the so-called HER2/neu oncogene as a driver in a subset of human breast cancer. This gene, which came to be known solely as the HER2 oncogene, was found to be "activated" in breast cancer as a result of a gene amplification event in the q14 region of chromosome 17 (17q14) (Borg et al. 1991; Berns et al. 1992; Kallioniemi et al. 1992; Liu et al. 1992). A number of studies showed conclusively that this gene amplification event resulted in high level overexpression of the HER2 gene at both the messenger RNA and protein level that was sufficient to transform breast epithelial cells to a malignant phenotype. Further studies demonstrated that inhibition of the kinase activity of this oncoprotein could result in growth inhibition of cancer cells bearing the amplification event as well as regression of HER2 driven breast cancers growing in immunodeficient mice. This work laid the groundwork for the ultimate development of the second targeted drug for breast cancer. (The first targeted drug for breast cancer, called Tamoxifen, inhibits the action of the estrogen receptor (ER). Much more on this later.) This FDA-approved drug, originally called Herceptin, is now known as Trastuzumab. Clinical studies using Trastuzumab, first in patients with HER2-amplified metastatic breast cancer, and later in the adjuvant setting, showed clearly that HER2 is a driving oncogene in most breast cancer patients with the HER2 amplification event, and that blocking the kinase activity of the oncoprotein has profound effects on progression and survival of HER2-positive breast cancer (Cobleigh et al. 1998; Slamon et al. 1998; Palmieri, Powles, and Vigushin 2001; Swain et al. 2015). Interestingly, while the HER2 protein is also a kinase, much like ABL, Trastuzumab doesn't work like Gleevec. That is, it is not a small molecule that fits into the enzymatic groove of the protein. Rather, because the HER2 protein is large and has a big chunk of the molecule that sticks outside of cells, Trastuzumab is an antibody molecule that binds to the extracellular parts of the HER2 protein and in that way, prevents its activation. It also now seems to be the case that because this drug is a humanized monoclonal antibody that targets the HER2 protein, immunological effects associated with the drug may also play a role in its effectiveness.

These two early success stories had an important feature in common: both drugs were found to be effective when targeting a genomically altered oncogene. That is, a gene that had acquired altered biological activity as a result of either a gene translocation event, or a gene amplification event. This commonality led to the assumption that became the basis for the development of many other targeted drugs in subsequent years. The assumption was that the product of any genomically altered driving oncogene would be a good target for a new drug, which would then be effective in patients with the specific oncogenic alteration. In some cases, these assumptions turned out to be correct. For example, we now have drugs (erlotinib, gefitinib, and Osimertinib) that are effective in lung cancer patients in which a driving oncogenomic alteration is an activating point mutation in a gene known as EGFR (Lynch et al. 2004; Shepherd et al. 2005; Tsao et al. 2005; Riely et al. 2006; Galvani et al. 2013). We also have a drug (vemurafenib) that is effective in patients with malignant melanoma in which a point mutation in the BRAF oncogene is the driving genomic alteration (Heakal, Kester, and Savage 2011; E.J. Jordan and Kelly 2012; Ravnan and Matalka 2012; Sharma et al. 2012). More recently, we have a drug (Alpelisib, among others) that appears to be effective in breast and other cancers in which a point mutation in a gene known as PIK3CA is the oncogenic driver (Armaghani and Han 2020; Copur 2020). These successes, which have had an impact on the standard of care for several cancer types, were consistent with the theory of oncogene addiction. Not surprisingly then, since as I mentioned earlier, there may be as many as 500 genes that play a role in cancer when they are activated as oncogenes, many other drugs have been developed and tested in the laboratory and in patients in which presumed activated oncogenes have been present. Unfortunately, many of these more recent clinical studies have not been as encouraging and many of these new drugs did not result in significant benefit for patients. These more recent results have tempered the early enthusiasm for the use of targeted drugs for cancer and the hope that they could one day replace traditional chemotherapeutic drugs.

So then, why don't targeted cancer drugs work better? And how do we do better at predicting those drugs that will be effective, and in which patients they will work best in? I once had a professor in graduate school who would say, "If the results of the experiment you perform are consistently different from what was predicted based on the hypothesis, then you should examine the assumptions that the hypothesis is based on". As we will see, this admonition is relevant to the question of why targeted drugs aren't more effective in patients with cancer than expected or predicted.

Gene essentiality as a predictor of good drug targets. The original use of the word "oncogene" was in the context of a gene that, when either overexpressed, or altered in its expression/activity because of some genomic event (translocation, amplification, point mutation) results in the *transformation* of a normal cell to one that expresses one of several transformed phenotypes relevant to cancer. The transformed phenotypes that were considered relevant to the malignant transformation process include immortalization (yes, cancer cells, unlike normal cells, can live forever!), growth factor independence, motility, invasion, and resistance to cell death (Hanahan and Weinberg 2000, 2011). Thus, oncogenes are considered drivers of the malignant phenotypes exhibited by cancer cells, and this notion has certainly stood the test of time. Here then is a case where an assumption was made about oncogenes that we are finding is not always correct. That assumption is that an oncogenic driver gene expressed in cancer cells is also a gene that is *essential* to the proliferation and survival of the cancer cells. The term essential, or essentiality, is critical here because if a driving oncogene is indeed essential to the proliferative potential or survival of the cancer cell, then it naturally would make a good drug target. Blocking the activity of such an essential gene would be highly detrimental to cancer cells but have little or no effect on normal cells. As we have seen, there are several oncogenes that meet this definition and are, indeed, good drug targets. But as we will see later, there are other genes that are considered to be bone fide oncogenes that turn out not to be good targets at all because even though they may be transforming, they are not always essential for the proliferation or survival of the cancer cells. We will discuss later how this can be true. In addition, we will also see that even in cases where a driver oncogene is a good drug target that is sometimes essential to the survival of the cancer cells, not all patients with the driver mutations will be sensitive to the targeted drugs. Thus, we have two separate but related problems that need to be solved if we are to improve our ability to use targeted cancer drugs in patients.

Now the question arises, how do we identify essential genes in cancer cells in an unbiased manner and figure out which oncogenes are truly essential? Also, might some cancer cells express other genes that are not actually oncogenes but are still essential in the cancer cells? If so, would these genes/proteins be good drug targets too?

To address this question, many research groups in academia and biotechnology have adopted strategies that can identify on a genome-scale all the essential genes in cancer cells. These screens provide functional data to otherwise descriptive genomic data that we have been accumulating on cancer cells and patients for many years now. For example, we now have access to large data sets from cancer patients that tell us, for individual patients, which and how many genes are amplified and overexpressed in their cancers (https://www.cancer.gov/about-nci/organization/ccg/research/ structural-genomics/tcga). These data sets are essentially descriptive in nature. While helpful, purely descriptive data has relatively little power because we know that the majority of these gene amplification events are passenger events that do not contribute to the pathogenesis of the disease experienced by the patient. As it turns out, because of the significant level of genomic instability in cancer, many if not most of the genomic changes that are detectable in cancer cells are not driver events, but passenger events. That is, the passenger events were acquired randomly and do not contribute to the pathogenesis of the disease. As a result, passenger genomic alterations in cancer cells result in significant noise in the descriptive genomic data available to us. Thus, while the technology that has been used to generate these types of descriptive genomic data sets are impressive, their power and impact for patients is limited. But, if we had a way to determine, on a gene by gene basis, which of those dozens to hundreds of gene amplification events (or mutation events or translocation events) were actually drivers of the disease progression, and if we had a way to determine which of those the cancer cells rely on for their behavior as cancer cells, then we would have powerful information that could be used to develop novel therapeutic strategies. That type of *functional* data can enhance the power and impact of the descriptive genomic data and transforms cancer genomics into Functional Genomics. As it happens, we do have such methods and these methods have been applied to hundreds of cancer cell lines derived from patients. These methods will be described in detail in Chapter 5. In the remainder of this book, I will argue that the functional genomic data that are currently available as a result of these extensive studies are the lynch pin for making strides against metastatic cancer in patients. But the key phrase that I just used in making this argument; *cancer cell lines derived from patients*, turns out to be fraught with a level of controversy and skepticism in the scientific community that has had a negative impact on the use of these kinds of data. Thus, before going into detail about how functional genomic data can be used to develop personalized targeted therapy strategies for cancer patients, I need to convince you first that the data that we currently have at our disposal that has been derived from cell lines, actually does reflect the real biology of cancer that is experienced by patients. So, let's give this a try.

CHAPTER 4

CELL LINES ARE PEOPLE TOO

So far in this book, I have described in fairly general terms how progress in cancer research over the decades has improved our ability to prevent cancers by understanding the biology of carcinogenesis in humans, and I have laid the groundwork for how obtaining a deeper understanding of cancer genomics, and particularly functional genomics, can provide new insights into the use of targeted cancer drugs. In the remainder of this book, I want to become much more specific and lay out a strategy that, I will argue, can lead to better uses of targeted cancer drugs that can ultimately have an impact on treatment of patients with metastatic disease.

To do that, I now need to focus the next several chapters on breast cancer specifically. For my nearly 40 years as a cancer researcher, I have studied the biology of breast cancer. Early in my career, my research focused on the factors that influence breast cancer progression in mouse models of breast cancer. Later, I turned my focus to rat models of breast cancer. When I started my career as an Assistant Professor at the University of Michigan Cancer Center, I turned my focus to human breast cancer, and kept that focus for the rest of my career. These breast cancer focused chapters will use actual data to demonstrate an overall strategy that will then be useable for any cancer type.

The central focus of the next chapters is the use of breast cancer cell lines in breast cancer research and the translation of that research to improve patient outcomes. I have developed a companion for this book called the Breast Cancer Cell Line Knowledge Base (SLKBase) and much of what I will outline here can be found on this web-based Knowledge Base (https://sumlineknowledgebase.com/). The SLKBase is designed to enhance the power of breast cancer research carried out by scientists around the world. The scientific premise that underlies all of this is that breast cancer cell lines, and indeed all carefully developed cell lines derived from human cancers, are currently undervalued and have not yet been used to their full potential in ways that can be translated to patients. Thus, as a community, we have not done all that we can to leverage the knowledge obtained from cell line-based research to further the cause of improved cancer therapies, particularly for patients with metastatic disease. Thus, I contend that when breast cancer cell lines that have been developed and maintained with scientific rigor are used properly, they represent an important gateway to the development of truly personalized targeted therapeutics for breast and other cancers.

One of the great advantages of the large panel of breast cancer cell lines that are available to researchers is that these breast cancer cell lines have been deeply characterized at many levels. As a result of comparative genomic hybridization studies and more recently genomic sequencing studies, all cell lines have been characterized for gene copy number changes, including copy number gains and losses, and focal gene amplifications. In addition, all cell lines have been characterized by expression profiling at the mRNA and protein levels using several platforms so that the expression levels of all genes are known for all cell lines. Exome sequence analysis has been used to identify all the Single Nucleotide Polymorphisms (SNPs) and point mutations present in every cell line. More recently, the genomic data associated with each cell line has been *functionalized* as a result of genome-scale shRNA or CRISPR essentiality (there's that word again) screens that have been carried out in a number of labs including my own. These screens have identified the most essential genes in each cancer cell line (https://depmap.org/portal/). This knowledge coupled with the recent extensive analysis of drug sensitivity across hundreds of targeted drugs for all breast cancer cell lines (https://www.cancerrxgene.org/) have yielded unparalleled data on the vulnerabilities of individual breast cancer cell lines. These vulnerabilities when analyzed in the context of the genomic profiling studies described above provide a gateway to the development of individualized approaches that can be used to reverse engineer individual cell lines. It is the ultimate goal of this work to use these strategies and apply them to individual breast cancer patients, particularly those with metastatic disease, as a way to develop truly personalized and precise strategies for best use of targeted cancer drugs.

If we are to take full advantage of the wealth of descriptive and functional data that have been obtained using breast cancer cell lines, we must start by changing the way they are viewed by some in the research community. We need to stop lumping cell lines together into groups, and instead, we must analyze each cell line as a patient. This, surprisingly enough, is a radical notion; that a particular breast cancer cell line is best thought of as a model of the disease experienced *by the patient* from which the cell line was developed. This approach is the key to developing truly personalized therapeutic approaches for cancer therapy, because if we can learn how to effectively reverse engineer dozens to hundreds of individual cell lines, then computational and machine learning methods can be used that will allow us to extrapolate those strategies to patients that share the same genomic features as the cell line. If we are to achieve this goal, I must first convince the reader that more work, not less, is needed using cancer cell lines derived from patients, as the functional genomic data currently available for these cell lines is the gateway to novel and personalized therapeutic strategies for cancer, particularly metastatic disease. Given that, let us start this section with a general discussion about the usefulness of breast cancer cell lines, and whether they are good models of human breast cancer as it occurs in patients.

What is a breast cancer cell line? "What is a breast cancer cell line" seems like an odd way to begin this section, but as I hope to convince you, it's a question that requires further discussion so that everyone has the same starting point for thinking about cell lines as models of individual human disease. Technically, we all know what a breast cancer cell line is; it's a continuously growing, immortal population of cells, breast cancer cells, that were isolated from a patient at some point, that have been growing in the lab ever since because they are, in fact, immortal. Because they are cancer cells, we know that they are most likely to be genomically abnormal. For many researchers, cell lines are useful because they have one or two defining characteristics that fall within the interest of the investigator or the lab in which they are being studied. For example, as we will see, there is an enormous literature that focuses on the biology of the estrogen receptor in breast cancer. And the vast majority of the work on estrogen receptor signaling in breast cancer has been carried out using a single cell line (MCF-7) because these breast cancer cells express a functional estrogen receptor. Most researchers who work in this area know little or nothing about the patient from which MCF-7 was derived and the state of disease experienced by the patient when the sample were procured. As a result, the cells are often viewed as little more than a useful laboratory tool. One of the negative and unintended consequences of this view is that, because cell lines like MCF-7 are easy to work with and are immortal, investigators can share the cells with other labs that have similar interests. After all, the cells can grow indefinitely, so one can actually farm them in the lab and distribute them all over the world. They are easy to freeze in a viable state, and thus they are easy to transport. One clear advantage of this strategy is that many labs in disparate parts of the world can perform research using cells from the same patient. What could go wrong? As we will see; plenty!

This description of a breast cancer cell line is one that would be shared by most cancer researchers who study breast cancer, particularly those that use in vitro models to study the disease. However, I will now argue, that this idea of what a breast cancer cell line is, is too narrow, resulting in negative consequences that have been counterproductive to breast cancer research.

So, let's begin again. A breast cancer cell line is derived from a patient. We all know that but unfortunately, it's not something most researchers think about very often. Let me give you an example of why we should, and how not thinking about this has had a negative impact on breast cancer research.

The development of the MCF-7 cell line. During the 1970s, the Michigan Cancer Foundation (MCF) located in Detroit Michigan was a hot bed of breast cancer research. There were pioneering breast cancer scientists there led by Dr. Gloria Heppner, and scientists such Fred and Bonnie Miller, Jose and Irma Russo, Charles McGrath, Charles King, Sam Brooks, and Jerome Horwitz (the developer of AZT but that's another story) to name a few. Also at that time, a little-known scientist named Herbert Soule was busy developing methods to culture breast cancer cells and normal breast epithelial cells from patients. Dr. Soule was a brilliant cell culturist, and a pioneer in the field, and as you may have surmised by now, he is the person who developed the MCF-7 breast cancer cell line (H. D. Soule et al. 1973) (later, Dr. Soule also developed the MCF-10A cell line series, and the lesser known MCF-12 cell line (H.D. Soule et al. 1990)). Dr. Sam Brooks was an endocrinologist who worked both at the MCF and at Wayne State University and is the person who determined that MCF-7 cells express a functional estrogen receptor.

The Founder and President of the Michigan Cancer Foundation was a man named Michael Brennan. Dr. Brennan was an oncologist as well as Director of the Myer L. Prentis Comprehensive Cancer Center of Metropolitan Detroit. It was his patient from whom the MCF-7 cell line was developed. Keep in mind, this was the 1970s, before the development of Tamoxifen, and the standard of care for patients with estrogen receptor positive breast cancer was oophorectomy as a form of hormonal therapy. Dr. Brennan's patient, a Catholic nun, by the way, did undergo oophorectomy along with her radical mastectomy. When the patient recurred with a pleural effusion *metastasis* Dr. Brennan began procuring those samples and providing them to Dr. Soule's lab. There were several such pleural effusion specimens brought to the lab, and Dr. Soule finally successfully propagated the cells that would become the MCF-7 cell line from a specimen procured six months before the patient died of her *metastatic* disease. Now, think about that sentence; the cell line was derived from cells procured from a pleural effusion metastasis of a patient with end stage breast cancer. As we will see, the lack of knowledge regarding the patient from which the most studied breast cancer cell line the world was procured is important and has resulted in a lot of well carried out but poorly interpreted research using this cell line.

From the perspective of the patient history, and particularly with the benefit of hindsight and knowledge gained from decades of subsequent breast cancer research, it would be straight forward to come to a few important conclusions about MCF-7 cells. The first conclusion is that this patient had estrogen receptor positive breast cancer. Nowadays patients with this type of disease are treated either with Tamoxifen, with Fulvestrant, or with aromatase inhibitors such as anastrozole. It is possible that this patient would have lived much longer had she had access to modern therapies for ER-positive breast cancer. Indeed, Tamoxifen was developed using MCF-7 cells and MCF-7-derived xenografts as the primary model system for development of this and other similar drugs. Interestingly, and importantly for the proper interpretation of data, MCF-7 cells only form tumors in immunodeficient mice when the animals are supplemented with estradiol. No estrogen, no tumors. For years after the development of the cell line, Abbot laboratories marketed their clinical ER test kit using MCF-7 cells as the control sample. In those days, clinical ER tests were performed using a biochemical binding assay, and estrogen binding to the ER of the MCF-7 cells was the gold-standard for this test. So, from all of this, it is clear that MCF-7 cells are a model for *metastatic*, estrogen receptor positive, estrogen-dependent breast cancer.

Unfortunately, many breast cancer researchers who work with this cell line have a different view because they have no idea of the patient history and the development of the cell line. Again, for many, MCF-7 is little more than a convenient laboratory tool because the cells express a functional estrogen receptor. As a result, many people who work with this cell line argue that MCF-7 cells are non-invasive and non-metastatic! These assumptions are based on interpretation of laboratory data with little or no appreciation for the patient data. How would so many people come to this conclusion? As it happens, for many scientists the only relevant measure of the ability of cancer cells to be invasive is their ability to invade artificial matrices in the laboratory. MCF-7 cells (like most luminal breast cancer cells) behave poorly in this assay. Similarly, for most researchers, the only determinant of the metastatic capacity of breast cancer cells is their ability to form either spontaneous or experimental metastases when injected into mice. Once again, like most luminal breast cancer cells, MCF-7 cells do not score in these mouse-based laboratory assays. Thus, most breast cancer scientists are comfortable with the laboratory data and know nothing of the clinical data and the patient history.

This makes no sense, and this incorrect idea has had a significant negative impact on research using this cell line. Do we really believe that data from experiments involving immune-deficient mice or artificial invasion assays are more relevant to the biology of the cells than data from the actual patient? This question and the debate that surrounds it are of great importance to the field because so much of the work that has been done with this cell line is based on important assumptions about the biology of the cells that, I would argue, are incorrect. Thus, the interpretation of the results of many of these experiments are also flawed. Over the years I have read many papers and attended many seminars in which the definitive statement that MCF-7 cells are a model of non-invasive, non-metastatic breast cancer cells is the starting point. As a result, the literature is filled with descriptions of experiments in which scientists are trying to *transform* MCF-7 cells into cells that are invasive in laboratory assays and metastatic in mice. These experiments, from the perspective of the true biology of MCF-7 cells and the biology of metastasis as it occurred in the patient, make absolutely no sense. And because of that, they are experiments that have been well carried out, and yet shed little light on the biology of breast cancer as it occurs in people, particularly metastatic ER-positive breast cancer.

Development the SUM series of human breast cancer cell lines. My perspective on cancer cell lines was shaped by work that I started when I was a post-doctoral fellow at the Michigan Cancer Foundation. The work I carried out at the MCF formed the basis of my later work that I carried out after joining the faculty of the University of Michigan. While at the MCF, I spent several years working with rat models of mammary carcinogenesis and as part of that work, my laboratory developed culture conditions for the long-term growth and serial passage of normal rat mammary epithelial cells, and then used that experience to begin developing culture methods for the long-term growth and development of cell lines from DMBA-induced rat mammary carcinomas (Ethier 1985, 1986). That experience was valuable, not only because it gave me and my lab a lot of hands-on experience working with primary cells from both normal and neoplastic tissues, but more importantly, because the work provided our first insight into the importance of growth factor independence as an *in vitro* phenotype associated with malignant potential *in vivo* (Ethier and Cundiff 1987). Those findings were the springboard for all our subsequent work on the mechanisms by which the HER2 oncogene regulates expression of transformed phenotypes in rodent breast cancer cells. In addition, the mechanistic connection between growth factor independence and malignant potential is what ultimately led to the development of culture conditions for the growth of human breast cancer cells in vitro, and the development of the SUM breast cancer cell lines in my laboratory.

The reason I know so much about the origins of the MCF series of cell lines is because I did my post-doctoral fellowship at the Michigan Cancer Foundation and spent five years there before moving on to an Assistant Professor position at the University of Michigan. During the five years I spent at the MCF, I had the opportunity to get to know Dr. Herbert Soule and I worked closely with him on several projects. In fact, I was there working right next door to him when he developed the MCF-10A cell line. Herb and I shared a New England heritage which helped with our personal relationship, because Herb could be a bit cantankerous.

In 1988 I left the MCF to join the faculty at University of Michigan in Ann Arbor, and in leaving the MCF, Herb was kind enough to give me frozen samples of several cell lines he'd been working with, including the newly developed MCF-10A and MCF-12 lines. One of the goals that I set for myself in starting my career at the University of Michigan was to make the transition from rodent models of breast cancer to human models. I had become very interested in growth factor independence in breast cancer and I wanted to extend our work into human cells. But a major limiting factor for that kind of work was the necessity to work with cells under growth-factor defined culture conditions, as we had done with the rat cells. All of the cell culture methods we had developed for normal and neoplastic rat mammary cells were growth factor supplemented media that also contained fetal bovine serum. Some of our media formulations contained very low serum levels or were serum-free and contained a series of hormones and growth factors. We spent several years working out the influence of each of those hormones and growth factors and their combinations on the proliferative potential of these cell types. Knowing that, it was discouraging to realize that all the human breast cancer cell lines that had been developed up to that time were developed and cultured under *undefined* conditions, usually consisting of some basal medium and 10% fetal bovine serum. What's more, the human breast cancer cell lines that everyone in the field worked with had been growing in these poorly defined conditions for many years, including MCF-7 cells. So, it quickly became clear to me that if I wanted to perform the kind of experiments with human breast cancer cells that I had done with rat mammary epithelial cells and rat mammary carcinoma cells, I would have to start working with primary cells myself.

Fortunately, my department chair at that time was Dr. Allen Lichter, a radiation oncologist whose clinical interest was in breast cancer. Allen was instrumental in setting up one of the first multi-disciplinary cancer clinics at the U of M Cancer Center, and when I told Allen what my goals were for my research in his department, he invited me to start attending the Monday multidisciplinary tumor board meetings. It was there that I met the surgical oncologists and medical oncologists who were the gate keepers when it came to procuring breast cancer tissue for my experiments. Nothing that I accomplished in the development of human breast cancer cell lines would have been possible without the enthusiastic support of Dr. Lichter, Dr. David August, Dr. Vern Sondak, Dr. Rob Cote, and many others. These oncologists enthusiastically embraced my research interest and made it possible for me to procure hundreds of breast cancer specimens from patients over the next several years, which ultimately resulted in the development of the SUM breast cancer cell line panel. At this point, I want to give a special acknowledgement to Dr. Barbara Weber for her role in helping me develop the SUM cell lines. I first got to know Barbara when she was doing her Medical Oncology Fellowship at Michigan and I was there when she joined the faculty to start her research career. It was Barbara who encouraged me to apply for the first ever Department of Defense breast cancer grant. During the first year of that program, the DOD had a special category for infrastructure grants that were aimed at developing breast cancer biobanks as shared resources and new model systems. I probably would not have applied for that grant without her encouragement, but I did apply, and received five years of support for the project that ultimately led to the development of the SUM cell line panel, and a bank of hundreds of specimens that were used by researchers at the University of Michigan and elsewhere. Given the work that the tissue bank supported and the fact that hundreds of labs have worked with the SUM breast cancer cell lines resulting in over 2000 publications, this grant mechanism was incredibly productive and has had a large impact on our field.

As a result of all this activity, which occurred within the first year or two of me joining the faculty at Michigan, my lab began working with breast cancer specimens that we procured from patients. As I mentioned earlier, I arrived at Michigan with cells that had been given to me by Herb Soule, and all these cells had an "MCF" designation. So, as we started to isolate and work with cells from the U of M patients, I needed to call them *something* that would distinguish them from the MCF cells I brought with me. And so, one day, in what was a rather light moment in the lab, we decided that the cells from tissues derived from U of M patients would become Steve's University of Michigan cells, and hence, the term SUM breast cancer cells was established. It was just a joke at first, but the name stuck, and here we are.

As I indicated at the beginning of this chapter, the companion to this book is the SUM Breast Cancer Cell Line Knowledge Base (SLKBase) (www.sumlineknowledgebase.com). The content that I put onto this Knowledge Base is based on my view that what we understand about the patient from whom a cell line was derived is critically important to understanding the cell line itself. Because of how important I consider it to be for scientists working with breast cancer cell lines to know the patient history and the type of disease they'd experienced, each of the SUM lines has a home page on the website that contains, among other things, a narrative summary of the development of each cell line. The narrative summaries tell everything that I know about the patient from whom the cells were isolated, and I tell everything that I know about each cell line based on my own work with the cells, the extensive data sets that we have generated with each cell line, and a summation of the published literature on each cell line. This, I hope, will be the starting point that will allow anyone working with any of the SUM cells to take a more holistic approach and work toward developing strategies that can effectively reverse engineer the malignant potential, or the survival, of the cells from each of these cell lines. In more recent updates to the SLKBase, I have provided the same types of data and information for 50 additional breast cancer cell lines. As I have implied earlier, I believe that a cell line should never be viewed solely as a laboratory tool, but rather as a surrogate for a patient with a specific type of disease. And thus, the more we understand about a given breast cancer cell line, the more we understand about the disease that the patient had when the sample was obtained.

All of this leads me to the key assumption that underlies the generation of the Knowledge Base, and which will be developed in detail in this book. That is, by developing a deep understanding of individual breast cancer cell lines, we should be able to figure out how to reverse engineer each cell line so that it is either no longer malignant, or no longer viable, in a manner that is specific to that cell line. And, if we can do that, we should be able to use that cell line to define identify patients represented by that cell line(s), and for whom that knowledge ought to be translatable. Achieving this lofty goal will require a systems approach or a more holistic approach to understanding breast cancer cell lines. Unfortunately, this approach is at odds with the more reductionist approach that most of the research community has taken over the decades. When you think about it, it's amazing that we can't already do this in a manner that is translatable. I think it's time we do better.

Breast Cancer Cell Lines as stable models of individual human disease. Breast cancer cell lines have been a mainstay of breast cancer research for decades. But even though many thousands of papers have been published describing data derived from the use of breast cancer cell lines (nearly 10,000 using MCF-7 cells alone!) there are some who now feel that cell lines are obsolete because they are poor models of the human disease. As a result, several groups have argued that alternative strategies are now needed to move the field forward and this has resulted in the promotion of organoid models and PDX models of breast cancer as superior ways to advance the field. And, while I would never argue that we shouldn't always be trying to find the best tools and strategies to perform breast cancer research, I think it's important that we not throw the baby out with the bath water and disregard or diminish the importance of cell line-based research based on scanty evidence that the lines don't adequately model human disease. So, at this point, I want to summarize the evidence in support of the use of breast cancer cell lines as valuable resources and argue that we have not done enough to fully leverage the power of breast cancer cell lines to understand the many types of human breast cancer and to identify their vulnerabilities.

To make the case that breast cancer cell lines are stable models of human disease, I'd like to start by recounting the time and circumstances when I first started to understand that breast cancer cell lines are, in fact, remarkably stable in their phenotypes and characteristics, when used properly. As I indicated earlier, during my post-doctoral fellowship at the Michigan Cancer Foundation in Detroit, I worked to develop cell culture media and methods for the growth and serial passage of normal rat mammary epithelial cells, and then cells from primary rat mammary carcinomas derived from DMBA-induced mammary tumors (Ethier and Moorthy 1991). Later, after joining the University of Michigan faculty, I worked to apply those cell culture media and methods to the growth of normal human mammary epithelial cells derived from reduction mammoplasties, and to primary human breast cancer cells. In pursuing this work, I quickly learned that the media I had developed for the rat cells worked well for normal human mammary epithelial cells (HME) cells, but these same media and methods were ineffective at growing breast cancer cells from patient specimens. Other groups, most notably the Martha Stampfer group at Berkeley and the Ruth Sager group at Harvard, were encountering similar problems using media that they had developed (Stampfer, Hallowes, and Hackett 1980; Hammond, Ham, and Stampfer 1984; Papadimitriou et al. 1989). As a result, we and others worked to modify our methods in an attempt to determine what it would take to successfully grow human breast cancer cells from patient samples on a routine basis. This work was being carried out in the late 1980s, and during that time, evidence was emerging that showed that the expression of intermediate filament proteins specific to epithelial cells, namely the cytokeratins, could be used to identify the lineage of different types of epithelial cells. Based on this work, it was found that most breast cancer cells in patients (particularly estrogen receptor positive cells) were of the luminal lineage, characterized by expression of cytokeratins 18 and 19 (Papadimitriou et al. 1989). These discoveries prompted my lab and others to examine the types of human mammary epithelial cells that we were able to culture using the methods we were using at that time. The answer was disappointing in that it became clear that the cell culture media that our lab and other labs were using would only support the growth of basal mammary epithelial cells, characterized by expression of cytokeratin 14, and did not support the growth of luminal mammary epithelial cells.

Based on these lineage-based observations, we realized that cell lines like MCF-7 and T47D, expressed the profile of luminal breast epithelial cells even after being in culture over 20 years. And these cell lines continued to express a functioning estrogen receptor. This then, was my first realization that the media and conditions used to isolate and culture human breast cancer cells from patient specimens has an impact on the cells that we can grow, and that when we get the conditions right, cells like MCF-7, which came from the pleural effusion metastasis of a patient with end-stage metastatic breast cancer, are remarkably stable for decades. To this day, MCF-7 cells exhibit the same luminal cytokeratin profile that they started with, and still express a functional estrogen receptor. Thus, once again, when properly maintained and cultured, MCF-7 represents a highly stable model of estrogen receptor positive metastatic breast cancer.

The dangers of sharing cell lines across laboratories. A quick aside is relevant to the story at this point. Many years ago, I reviewed a paper for Breast Cancer Research and Treatment in which MCF-7 cells had been obtained from several laboratories around the world and tested in a single lab for characteristics of true MCF-7 cells. As one might have predicted, the characteristics observed in the cells obtained from different labs varied widely. In my assessment of this paper, I wanted to determine how the phenotypes of the "MCF-7" cells in different laboratories related to the provenance of each of the cell lines. This was a natural question for me having once worked with Dr. Soule at the MCF. What I discovered was that any cell line that I could trace directly (one degree of separation) back to the MCF exhibited the proper morphology, estrogen receptor expression, and other phenotypes of MCF-7 cells. By contrast, the cells that investigators had obtained from laboratories other than the originating lab, varied widely in their phenotypes and many no longer expressed the estrogen receptor. We now know as a result of the recent use of STR profiling (DNA finger printing like that used by modern law enforcement) of cell lines, is that this kind of inter-lab "variability" is not the result of instability, but rather the result of poor cell culture technique and sharing of cell lines across laboratories. So, if MCF-7 cells in a laboratory no longer express the estrogen receptor, it is likely because they are actually Hela cells, or some other common contaminant, rather than *bone fide* MCF-7 cells. Hela cells were derived from the cervical carcinoma of a patient once thought to be named Helen Lane. However, we now know that the patient that the cells were derived from was Henrietta Lacks and this story has now been widely told (Skloot 2011). The point is that HeLa cells are so proficient at growth in the laboratory that they have come to contaminate many cell lines leading people to think they are working with cells lines like MCF-7 (a breast cancer cell line) when they are really working with HeLa cells (a cervical cancer cell line).

The take home lesson from this is clear; one should never-ever obtain a cell line from anyone who isn't the original source of the cells, or at the very least, has a first-degree connection to that original source. And STR validation should always be done with any cell line that comes into a lab. To do otherwise is to put the research carried out in that lab at risk. And yes, this means investigators actually have to purchase the cells to be used in the experiments. Isn't the integrity of research worth a few hundred dollars? Most labs happily pay hundreds to thousands of dollars to purchase a tube of an antibody that gets used up and must be purchased again. Cell line purchases are a one-time thing and provides the lab with a stable and reliable resource for decades. If we are to maintain rigor in cell line-based research, scientists must stop getting cells from friends or neighboring labs. This practice is one of the main reasons for the demonstrated lack of rigor and reproducibility that has been much publicized in recent years and has contributed mightily to the mistaken notion that cell lines are inherently unstable (Freedman, Gibson, Ethier, et al. 2015; Freedman, Gibson, Wisman, et al. 2015). This is an easy and inexpensive problem to solve.

Okay, back to our story. Based on observations of lineage and estrogen receptor stability in MCF-7 and other cell lines, we set out to modify our culture media and conditions in a way that would allow us to culture luminal breast epithelial cells from normal tissue. We reasoned that being able to culture normal luminal mammary epithelial cells would result in more success in growing breast cancer cells from patients. In some ways, the modifications that we made to accomplish this goal were remarkably simple. In other ways, these modifications led us to discover still other barriers to the successful culture of breast cancer cells from patient samples. On the positive side, we discovered fairly quickly that simply adding 5% fetal bovine serum to the otherwise more complex growth factor supplemented serum-free media that we used to successfully culture basal mammary epithelial cells, resulted in excellent proliferation of cells with a distinct morphology in culture and which expressed high levels of cytokeratin 8, 18, and 19. Not long after, we discovered that the key growth factor present in serum that was responsible for the emergence and proliferation of luminal cells was lysophosphatidic acid (LPA). When we used our original serum-free formulation and then added LPA, we were able to routinely culture this second morphotype of mammary epithelial cells that expressed the luminal cytokeratins.

Armed with these two newer media formulations, we once again attempted to culture bone fide human breast cancer cells from patient derived primary tumors. At first, we thought we were successful as we were clearly able to culture luminal cells from primary breast cancers. The problem though, as we discovered after analyzing these cells for the genomic features of the breast cancer cells derived from the patients, and after measuring their proliferative lifespan in culture, was that what we had done is discovered a way to efficiently grow normal luminal mammary epithelial cells from breast cancer specimens, and not the breast cancer cells themselves. Indeed, we found that we could do this with every breast cancer specimen that we worked with. Two steps forward, one step back.

Thus, to directly test if our newly developed culture medium could support the growth of bone fide breast cancer cells, we decided to work with metastatic specimens, either from lymph nodes, pleural effusions, or skin metastases because these sites would be devoid of normal luminal mammary epithelial cells. Once again, this strategy resulted in good news and bad news, and in this case the bad news came first. We found that breast cancer cells from malignant pleural effusions from patients with metastatic breast cancer would not grow in our highly enriched culture medium. Furthermore, the cells were particularly unhappy on the collagen coated culture dishes that we had always used to grow normal cells. The good thing about working with cells from pleural effusion metastases though is that since some of these specimens yielded tens of millions of cancer cells that could be frozen directly, we could try many different media formulations on cells from the same patient. And, having started with a highly enriched culture medium that supported the growth of normal mammary epithelial cells but not breast cancer cells, we then did the only logical thing left, and that was to begin omitting factors one by one. Amazingly, the more factors we omitted, the better the cells did! First, omitting the collagen coating was helpful, but also omitting factors like epidermal growth factor (EGF) and the agents being used to boost cAMP levels in the cells, and even omitting the estrogen, progesterone and prolactin, all had positive effects on the growth of the metastatic cells. And, by simplifying the medium, we were also able to dramatically reduce the growth of unwanted stromal cells, or mesothelial cells in the case of pleural effusions. Interestingly, the success of these less complex media was consistent with our original hypothesis of the importance of growth factor-independence as an important phenotype of breast cancer cells.

This paired down growth medium allowed us to characterize two other important features of breast cancer cells. The first is that, unlike normal cells in highly enriched media which grow rapidly, primary breast cancer cells grow slowly with population doubling times on the order of 200 hours. This feature, as it happens, is entirely consistent with what was known about the kinetics of breast cancer growth in patients. Second, also unlike normal cells, primary breast cancer cells do not grow well at clonal densities and need to be maintained at high densities in culture. We followed up on this observation and found that the density dependence of breast cancer cells could be overcome by culturing breast cancer cells at clonal density in the presence of conditioned medium derived from high density cultures of the same cells! This in itself was not terribly surprising since at the time the autocrine hypothesis for growth factor independence had become well accepted. What was surprising, however, was our finding that the "factors" in condition medium that allowed cells to grow at low density were completely dialysable. That is, these were small molecules of the kind normally shared by cells via gap junctional intercellular communication. Around this time, work from Dr. James Trosko's laboratory at Michigan State University had shown that most breast cancer cells had lost the ability to communicate by GJIC as a result of down-regulation of certain connexins (Trosko and Ruch 1998). Thus, our observations were consistent with those findings.

Because it took quite some time for us to come to these realizations and conclusions, the very first breast cancer cell line developed in our lab is called SUM-44, because this was our first success after 43 tries! But, like MCF-7 cells, SUM-44 cells to this day, maintain their morphology, express luminal cytokeratins, and express very high levels of a functional estrogen receptor. SUM-44 cells exhibit the same characteristics they did in the patient and are stable when cultured in the medium used to isolate them (Ethier et al. 1990). In addition, SUM-44 cells, having been derived from a patient with infiltrating lobular carcinoma, exhibit a point mutation in the CDH1 gene (E-cadherin) that is a definitive feature of this type of breast cancer. And, when these cells are injected into the primary lactiferous duct of immunodeficient mice, they generate continuously growing breast cancers that exhibit the morphology of luminal breast cancer and resemble the histology of the patient specimen (Sflomos et al. 2021). Thus, SUM-44 cells are an excellent model of estrogen receptor positive, metastatic, lobular breast cancer. As a result, a rich literature has emerged in which these cells have been used as a model to understand this disease type better.

Over the years, evidence has mounted on many levels that supports the notion that cell lines, when properly cultured and maintained, are remarkably stable models of specific types of human breast cancers. This is particularly true at the level of the driving genomic alterations that are at the heart of the biology of the patient's disease. Several decades ago, the SKBR3 cell line was developed. These cells have a focal amplification of the 17q12 genomic region which is the genomic location of the HER2 oncogene. As a result, SKBR3 cells have a HER2 gene amplification and overexpress HER2 at the mRNA and protein level. These cells have been used by many investigators to study the biology of HER2 as a breast cancer oncogene and the cells have been used to develop the HER2 targeted therapies that are in routine use in the clinic today.

In the late 1990s we developed the SUM-190 and SUM-225 cells lines each of which also has a focal amplification of ERBB2 (HER2) with overexpression at the message and protein level, and which are responsive to HER2 targeted drugs. The SUM-225 cell line was derived from a patient who had a modified radical mastectomy for extensive high grade (comedo) ductal carcinoma *in situ* and then had a chest wall recurrence. We developed the cell line from the chest wall nodule, and when these cells are grown as xenografts in immune-deficient mice, the tumors that develop exhibit that same comedo growth pattern as seen in the original patient specimen and chest wall nodule (Behbod et al. 2009; Smith et al. 2022). Thus SUM-225 is an excellent of model of aggressive DCIS that maintains the genomic feature of the driving oncogene, and the same *in vivo* growth pattern that was observed in the patient. These properties of the SUM-225 cell line were first reported some 20 years ago (Shekhar et al. 2013) and this phenotype has been maintained over many years in culture.

The SUM-190 cell line, in addition to having a focal ERBB2 amplification, has a point mutation in the PIK3CA oncogene, which results in sensitivity of these cells to the class I-alpha specific drug Alpelisib. Interestingly, the PIK3CA mutation also results in reduced sensitivity of these cells to HER2-specific tyrosine kinase inhibitors (Guest et al. 2016). Like for the SUM-225 cells, these characteristics have not changed over the 20 years that we and others have been working with them. The story of HER2 amplification and the dependence on HER2 activity for their growth and survival in a number of breast cancer cell lines is yet another indication of the remarkable *stability* of the phenotypes of human breast cancer cell lines.

The SUM-149 (https://sumlineknowledgebase.com/?page_id=249) and SUM-190 (https://sumlineknowledgebase.com/?page_id=249) cell lines came from patients with inflammatory breast cancer, and both cell lines over express E-cadherin, which is a common characteristic of this type of breast cancer.

This cell line stability can be observed at many levels in addition to the driving oncogenes characteristic of each line. A number of years ago, Charles Perou and colleagues used unsupervised cluster analysis of the transcription profiles of primary cancer specimens and identified several molecular sub-types of breast cancer (Ross et al. 2000; Ross and Perou 2001; Prat, Adamo, et al. 2013; Prat, Karginova, et al. 2013). This work has been reproduced by many labs both at the mRNA and protein level and is considered established science in breast cancer. The Perou research group went on to demonstrate that breast cancer cell lines can be assigned to the same cluster groups as primary breast cancers based on unsupervised analysis of their expression profiles. This represents yet another strong line of evidence of the fidelity of breast cancer cell lines as models of specific types of breast cancer.

Even the morphology of breast cancer cells does not change over time as can be clearly seen from the very different morphologies of the SUM cells, which has not changed over the 20+ years I have been working with them.

I could go on but hopefully by now the point is made. Breast cancer cell lines, ***when properly obtained and properly cultured*** are highly stable models of the specific disease of the patient from which they came, and they maintain those characteristics over decades. Thus, breast cancer cell lines are people too!

By now, you may be wondering why I'm making such a big deal about this. The reason is this: if you accept that individual breast cancer cell lines are good and stable models of the disease that was experienced by the patient from which they came, then an enormous amount of omics-based data becomes available that can be used to enhance the meaning of cell line-based research. As a result of work from the Joe Gray lab, from project Achilles at Dana Farber, from the MD Anderson reverse phase protein array lab, from the Cell Line Encyclopedia and the Genomics of Drug Sensitivity in Cancer database developed by the Wellcome Sanger Institute, there is an enormous amount of data for over 70 breast cancer cell lines and for hundreds of other cancer cell lines derived from individual patients with cancer. These data can be used to move the field forward, particularly toward improving our ability to deliver precision therapeutics to patients. Thus, one of the goals of this book, and the SLKBase, is to make these data available to our users and readers in a way that yields deep biological insights into individual breast cancer cell lines as *individual patients*. Bringing these tools to our users will allow us to obtain a deeper understanding of cell lines, one patient at a time. Then, we can use that knowledge to generate novel strategies to reverse engineer each of these cell lines. Despite the emerging popularity of organoid models and PDX models of breast cancer, none of these experimental systems come with anywhere near the amount and sophistication of the data that we have for cell lines, nor are these systems amenable to the generation of these kinds of data sets, particularly gene essentiality studies. Moreover, they are not flexible enough to allow creative experimentation to be done to test predictions that result from the volumes of functional omics data we have for cell lines.

Apparent instability of breast cancer cell lines: In the paragraphs above, I've attempted to provide a brief summary of the evidence that points to the inherent *stability* of human breast cancer cell lines as models of human disease and the impact that this has had on breast cancer research. However, many will still argue that breast cancer cell lines are unstable. As a result, many researchers have turned away from using these models, and consider this instability to be a significant disadvantage. So, what are we to make of this apparent conflict?

There are two general explanations for "instability" that has been observed by researchers using breast cancer cell lines. One explanation isn't really an explanation at all because the instability that some have observed is more apparent than real and is the result of sloppy cell culture technique that results in contamination of one cell line with another. We've all heard the stories about the ubiquity of the HeLa cell line and many researchers have discovered to their horror that cells they've been using for years are not at all what they thought they were. Another less famous example of cell line contamination invalidating the results of experiments performed with them is the development and use of the so-called MCF-7/ADR cells. This cell line was for many years thought to be a drug resistant version of MCF-7 cells. But of course, these cells were not derived from MCF-7 cells at all, nor do they bare any resemblance to MCF-7 cells.

The use of experimental approaches to develop drug resistant variants by culturing cells for long periods of time in the presence of a drug and waiting for cells to emerge that can grow in the presence of the drug is ripe for the type of cell line contamination that occurred in the development of MCF-7/ADR. During the selection period, the vast majority of cells in the culture dish are killed by the drug treatment, and thus, if even a single clonogenic cell that happens to be more resistant to the drug then the original cell line, contaminates any of those culture dishes, the cells that will emerge will be the result of the contaminant, and not the selection of a drug resistant variant. So, if care is needed in the routine use of breast cancer cell lines, extreme care is needed if one is to use such a selection approach to develop variants from a parental cell line. STR profiling, therefore, should always be carried out to validate the origin of any drug-resistant variant cell line derived in culture.

The second explanation for the apparent "instability" of breast cancer cell lines is more interesting and more relevant to a key question in cancer biology. This problem and has to do, not with the instability of the cell lines, but of their inherent *heterogeneity*, which is present in all human cancers. The notion of cellular heterogeneity of breast cancer specimens and cell lines was pioneered by Drs. Gloria Heppner and Fred Miller of the Michigan Cancer Foundation (G.H. Heppner et al. 1978; G.H. Heppner et al. 1983; Miller, Miller, and Heppner 1984; G. Heppner et al. 1986). She and her colleagues at the MCF were the first to show that breast cancer specimens and cell lines are comprised of sub-populations of cells that vary in their growth potential, their tumorigenic potential, and their metastatic potential. This idea has stood the test of time and the study of heterogeneity of cancer is now one of the hottest topics in the field. So, in this regard, once again cell lines accurately mimic the real biology of breast cancer. As such, they can be used to identify, clone or isolate different sub-populations of cells within the cell line to understand the contribution that each sub-population makes to the overall malignant potential of the parental cell line. This is a feature and not a bug of breast cancer cell lines and allows for the study of the role of cancer cell heterogeneity in the biology of the disease. There are excellent papers in the literature in which sub-populations of cells were isolated from cancer cell lines and their individual contributions to the overall biology and malignant potential of the parent cell line was demonstrated (Brown et al. 2022; Naffar-Abu Amara et al. 2020).

The study of breast cancer stem cells is founded on the demonstrated ability to sort the stem cell population from a parental cell line using cell surface or biochemical markers of stem cells. Those isolated stem cells have been shown to regenerate the heterogeneity observed in the parental cell line (Dontu et al. 2003; Ginestier et al. 2007; Charafe-Jauffret et al. 2009). Thus, the so-called instability that some researchers worry about reflects the natural heterogeneity of breast cancers and breast cancer cell lines. Thus, breast cancer cell lines provide a powerful tool for the study of cellular heterogeneity in cancer. Of course, this complexity makes it even more critical that researchers work with cell lines with great care and rigor to avoid unwanted selection of sub-populations of cells so as not to mistake heterogeneity for instability.

In summary, I hope that I've convinced you that breast cancer cell lines are people too! As such, they continue to be relevant and powerful sources of knowledge on the biology of breast cancer. The recent elucidation of functional genomic data sets only deepens their importance and relevance to the human disease. In the chapters that follow, I will show how a functional genomic analysis of a large panel of breast cancer cell lines can lay the groundwork for the next generation of targeted therapeutic strategies for breast cancer, particularly for patients with metastatic disease. Since overt metastatic breast cancer remains incurable, much work still needs to be done to improve survival of patients with metastatic breast cancer.

CHAPTER 5

PUTTING THE FUNCTION IN FUNCTIONAL GENOMICS: RNA-INTERFERENCE AND CRISPR BASED SCREENS AS PREDICTORS OF GENE ESSENTIALITY

If after reading the previous chapter and you are still with me, and are willing to consider how we can make better use of cancer cell lines to predict the best drug targets and drug sensitivities in patients, then we now need to discuss the methods that we and others have used over the past several years to examine, on a gene by gene bases, the role or essentialness of individual genes in the proliferation and/or survival of cancer cell lines derived from hundreds of different patients.

The methods that I am about to describe were originally developed and pioneered by scientists at the Memorial Sloan Kettering and Dana Farber Cancer Centers, and are referred to as genome-scale essentiality screens (T. Wang et al. 2014; T. Wang et al. 2015; T. Wang, Lander, and Sabatini 2016; Gonen et al. 2017; Kim and Hahn 2007; Tsherniak et al. 2017). These powerful methods are best used in cancer cell lines, though there have been some attempts to use similar approaches in in vivo models of cancer, but with less power and success.

The basic approach to a gene essentiality screen is to use either RNA-interference approaches or CRISPR-based approaches to either knock down or knock *out* every expressed gene in the genome of a cancer cell line one-by-one and determine how the loss of expression of that gene influences the survival or proliferation of the cancer cells in the cell line. How, you may be wondering, is this possible?

The experimental approach involves the use of very large libraries of individual short-hairpin-RNA (shRNA) or CRISPR vectors that can be transduced into cells using viral carriers such that, when those constructs are expressed, they either reduce or eliminate the expression of the target gene. RNA-interference (RNAi) works be targeting sequences in the mRNA of specific genes and dramatically reducing (knocking down) the translation of those messages into protein. By contrast, CRISPR makes use of guide-RNA (sgRNA) vectors to seek out the DNA sequences of their target genes and damage them in a way that prevents, or knocks out, expression of the gene.

In the Ethier lab, we used an shRNA library consisting of over 81,000 shRNA vectors targeting over 15,000 well annotated human genes to perform gene essentiality screens for the SUM breast cancer cell line panel that I developed, as well as for MCF-7, MCF-7LTED, and MCF-10A cell lines (Turner-Ivey et al. 2014; Guest et al. 2015; Guest et al. 2016). The Hahn laboratory at the Dana Farber Cancer Center also performed shRNA (RNAi) screens on hundreds of cell lines, some of which are breast cancer lines. The Hahn lab also performed CRISPR based screens on many cell lines and there is considerable overlap in the list of cell lines for which screen data are available from both types of screens. Other groups have also performed these types of genome-scale essentiality screens on several cancer cell lines.

As I indicated above, the shRNA library that we used contains over 81,000 separate lentiviral vectors that can target over 15,000 genes. This means that within the library, there are approximately 5 different shRNA constructs for each gene, with each shRNA designed to target a different part of the mRNA molecule. This redundancy is essential for proper interpretation of the data, as we will see. I mentioned that each shRNA construct is packaged in a lentivirus, and the use of this type of virus is critical to the success of the experiment. These lentiviral constructs are engineered so that the actual viruses that we make in the lab are harmless to people and act only as a vehicle to deliver the shRNA or CRISPR vector into the cells. There are two key aspects of how lentivirus work that make the experiment doable. First, once inside the cells, the viral RNA genome is reverse transcribed to generate a DNA-proviral copy and this piece of DNA then integrates randomly into the genome of the infected cell. By using these vectors, we effectively introduce a new gene into the genome of the cell the sole function of which is to either knock down or knock out its target gene. The second advantage of using lentiviral constructs instead of other types or retroviral constructs is that the infected cells can express the new gene without having to be in the S-phase of the cell cycle. So, essentially every cell that gets infected with the virus will generate the DNA-provirus that will then integrate into the host cell genome and then transcribe its RNA*i* (RNA-interference) or sgRNA (CRISPR) construct.

In generating the lentiviral library and then infecting the cells to be tested, two important parameters must be met. First, we want the library to contain between 1000 and 5000 copies of each of the 81,000 vectors. Thus, for each experiment, we transduce the cells to be tested with roughly 400 million viral particles. The second important parameter is the so-called multiplicity of infection (MOI). That is, if we transduced 400 million viral particles into 400 million cancer cells, we would have a MOI of 1. But what we want is an MOI of between 0.1 and 0.3 in order to make it unlikely that any cell gets infected with more than one viral particle, which is important for the clear interpretation of the result. Thus, we would take our 400 million virus prep and use it to infect approximately 1 billion cancer cells (this is getting to be a big experiment!). Now there are two other key aspects of lentiviral constructs that we use to build these libraries. One is the construct contains an antibiotic resistance gene that renders any cell that was successfully infected resistant to an antibiotic drug such as neomycin. This allow us to eliminate any cells from the population that were not infected leaving us with a starting population of cells all of which has been infected by just one viral particle. The second key factor is that each viral construct contains a "DNA bar code", a sequence of 12 nucleotides that is unique to each viral construct. As we will see, this is what actually gets measured in the essentiality experiment. As will also become evident, the advent of powerful DNA sequencing technology dramatically increased the power of these experiments.

Given all of that, here is how the experiment is carried out. First, the cell population is infected with the lentiviral library preparation, and this is the easy part. The next day, the antibiotic drug is added to the culture to kill off any uninfected cells. Two days after that, half of the infected cells are harvested, their DNA is isolated and then sequenced in a way that allows us to count the individual bar codes associated with each viral construct. This tells us the starting number of each shRNA or CRISPR construct in the population at the start of the experiment. Then, the remaining cells are cultured for one to two weeks so that the population of cells expands approximately 30 to 50 times. The cells are then harvested again and DNA isolated. Because each construct generates a pro-viral DNA copy that gets integrated into the host cell genome, every time a cell goes through the cell cycle and replicates its DNA, the proviral gene (and the bar code) also gets replicated. Now, imagine that a particular proviral gene codes for the expression of an shRNA molecule that targets a gene that is either not expressed in the cell, or is not essential to the cell's survival or proliferation. In that case, the expression of that shRNA will have no effect on the proliferation of the cells containing that provirus and thus the copy number of the bar code associated with that vector will also increase roughly 30 to 50 times over the course of the experiment (remember, roughly 1000 cells got infected with each vector). Thus, by performing a second DNA sequencing at the end of the experiment, we can count the bar codes and compare each to the starting number determined on day 3. By contrast, if the shRNA expressed in the cell targets and knocks down a gene that is critical for the cells to undergo cell proliferation, then the loss of that gene will prevent the cells from dividing over the course of the experiment. Thus, when we count the bar codes at the end of the experiment, the bar code number for this vector will have stayed roughly the same as it was at the beginning of the experiment. Finally, if the shRNA construct knocked down a gene that was essential to the *survival* of the cells infected then the number of those bar codes present at the end of the experiment will actually decrease during the experiment and so the bar code count will be less than it was at the beginning.

As you can see, this is an elegant and powerful experiment that makes use of the most modern methods of molecular biology and genomic sequencing. And, because each experiment generates enormous amounts of data, it requires elegant bioinformatic and statistical analysis to correctly interpret the data, and these too have been developed and refined over the years.

The result of all of this is a powerful data set that quantitatively describes the essentialness of every expressed gene in the genome of the cells tested. And, as will be shown next, this gene essentiality data adds functional significance to the other types of omic data that we have for these cancer cell lines.

Functionalizing Genomic Data using gene essentiality. As you can tell from the description of the gene essentiality experiments, the data output is a long list, over 15,000 genes long, of an essentiality value for every gene that was targeted by the library. Anyone who already has experienced looking at long lists of data generated from other types of omics studies understands how mind numbing and therefore uninformative these lists can be. Furthermore, if all one has are long lists of genes with associated pieces of data, they are highly subject to confirmation bias because the most natural thing for people to do is to scan the list looking for their favorite genes or genes whose name they recognize and focus only on the data associated with those genes, and basically ignore the rest. This is a very poor way to analyze these kinds of omics data sets. So, what's the alternative?

Enter orthogonal analysis of omics data sets. One of the bad things about large omics data sets derived from various types of sequencing of cancer cells is that they are noisy. That is, they contain a lot of data much of which is not informative. Thus, the signal to noise ratio can be quite small. But, by using gene essentiality data to orthogonally analyze other omics data sets, the essentiality data can be used to filter the data, which has the effect of dramatically increasing the signal to noise ratio and in that way, adding great biological significance to the data.

For example, we have genome-wide copy number/gene amplification data from hundreds of cancer cell lines and as we have described, gene amplification is one important mechanism by which oncogenes become activated. The problem, however, is that all gene amplification data sets are noisy because most of the amplified genes that are detected are the result of events that do not contribute directly to the malignant properties of the cancer cell. Such genomic changes in cancer cells are referred to as passenger events and are distinguished from driver events. So, how does one distinguish driver events from passenger events? It may be obvious by now that gene essentiality can be used to functionalize those copy number data and point us toward the small number of genes in which the amplification event had functional significance for the cancer cells. As we published in our OncoTarget paper (Guest et al. 2016), we used gene essentiality data derived from our shRNA-based screen of the SUM breast cancer cell lines to filter the gene amplification data we already had for our cell lines. To cite one example, the SUM-52 breast cancer cell line has hundreds of copy number alterations and amplified genes. However, when we only consider those genes that are amplified <u>and</u> overexpressed <u>and</u> essential as determined by the screen (orthogonal analysis of three data sets from the same cell line), we are left with an oncogene signature that consists of only 5 genes! By orthogonal analysis of copy number data, gene expression data and gene essentiality data we reduced the complexity of the data set over 100-fold resulting in a data set that is all or almost all signal and without significant noise. Furthermore, the result of this analysis is independent of whether we know anything about the genes that are found to be important and thus the result if free of confirmation bias. The cells and the data tell us the gene amplification events that are most important to the cancer cells. This same type of exercise can be carried out by analyzing gene essentiality data with respect to point mutation data or gene expression data which, once again, provides functional significance to those genomic events in cancer cells.

As a result of the essentiality screens we performed with the SUM cell lines, we were able to functionalize the other genomic data available to us and this had a profound impact on our understanding of the biology of the oncogenes present in these cells. For example, after we developed the SUM-185 cell line we used traditional methods in an attempt to identify the driving oncogenes in this cell line. Because these traditional methods focused on identification of known candidate oncogenes, we initially failed at determining the oncogene signature for this cell line. However, following array comparative genomic hybridization (CGH) analysis of this cell line, we identified a small amplicon on the telomeric portion of chromosome 4, which is the locus of the FGFR3 gene. We went on to show that FGFR3 was both amplified and overexpressed in these cells making it a strong candidate oncogene, despite the fact that FGFR3 amplification is rare in breast cancer. When we performed the shRNA screen on the SUM-185 cell line, the FGFR3 gene was a strong hit indicating that this amplified gene is essential to SUM-185 cells. And, as would be predicted based on the hypothesis that gene essentiality predicts drug sensitivity (to be discussed in detail later), SUM-185 cells are exquisitely sensitive to an FGFR targeted drug. This functional genomic analysis of SUM-185 cells also led to the discovery of another amplified oncogene, BCL2L1 which was also determined to be essential in the screen, and a point mutated oncogene PIK3CA also found to be essential. Once again, it turned out that SUM-185 cells are also exquisitely sensitive to Navitoclax, a drug that targets both BCL2 and BCL2L1, and Alpelisib, a drug that targets the type I alpha isoform of PI3'kinase, the product of the PIK3CA oncogene. Thus, the use of gene essentiality data to functionalize the other omic data from SUM-185 revealed a basic *functional oncogene signature* that correctly predicted exquisite drug sensitivity.

Similar experiments with SUM-225 cells confirmed the essentiality of ERBB2 (HER2), which is amplified and overexpressed in these cells. Experiments with the SUM-190 cell line revealed an unexpected finding that, as we will see, was also found in other ERBB2 amplified cell lines. SUM-190 cells have an amplification and overexpression of the ERBB2 (HER2) oncogene. In addition, these cells have a point mutation in the PIK3CA oncogene. It is well known that the HER2 oncogene is a tyrosine kinase that signals through the PI3'kinase pathway. Thus, SUM-190 cells have *redundant* genomic alterations; an amplified HER2 gene signaling through a pathway with a PIK3CA mutation. Interestingly, we found that in SUM-190 cells, HER2 did not score as an essential gene but PIK3CA did score as essential. When we examined these cells for sensitivity to HER2 or PIK3CA targeted drugs, we found that the cells were indeed highly sensitive to the PIK3CA targeted drug Alpelisib but were 10-fold more resistant to the HER2 targeted drug than the SUM-225 cells. Thus, once again, the shRNA essentiality screen correctly predicted the drugs to which the cells are most sensitive. In other SUM breast cancer cell lines, the shRNA screen identified mutant HRAS and KRAS oncogenes as drivers in two cell lines, and mutant PIK3CA oncogene as a functional driver in two additional SUM cells.

RNA-interference versus CRISPR based gene essentiality screens. As was mentioned at the outset of this chapter, different laboratories have performed genome-scale essentiality screens using either shRNA libraries or CRISPR libraries. So, what's the difference between RNAi and CRISPR-based screens and which method is better at predicting the cancer genes that are good drug targets?

Whereas the goal for each type of screen is the same and the basic experimental approach is the same, shRNA and CRISPR vectors operate in fundamentally different ways that must be kept in mind when interpreting the screen/essentiality data, particularly when thinking about how the results relate to druggability and drug sensitivity. shRNA screens work by knocking *down* the level of expression of the target gene at the mRNA level, whereas CRISPR screens work by knocking *out*, at the DNA level, the target of the guide RNAs. Thus, genes that are found to be essential and score as hits in the shRNA screens are those for which *reductions* in the levels of gene expression can have a significant effect on proliferation or survival of the cell line. By contrast, since the CRISPR screens work by knocking *out* the target gene, this approach identifies all genes that are essential when expression of the target gene is eliminated completely. As a result, the CRISPR approach tends to be more sensitive than the RNAi approach and identifies more essential genes in a given cell line because there are more genes that are essential when eliminated than when simply reduced in their expression. As a result of this fundamental difference, CRISPR screens also identify a larger number of *common essential* genes than those found in RNAi based screens. Common essential genes are defined as those genes that would score as essential in virtually any cell line tested (normal or cancer) because they perform a basic function that is essential to cell proliferation or survival in most if not all cells. Thus, if one is using screen data to identify vulnerabilities specific to individual cancer cell lines, identifying a gene in a screen that is commonly essential is not particularly informative for that cell line. Thus, the number of common essential genes identified using the two different methods differs significantly because there are many genes that, when reduced in expression, do not have a significant impact on proliferation or survival, but have a big impact when knocked out completely. A dramatic example of this effect can be seen by comparing the results of RNAi and CRISPR screens in common cell lines. For example, the Hahn lab performed a CRISPR screen on the SUM-159 cell line, and the Ethier lab analyzed this cell line using an shRNA library. The CRISPR screen pathway analysis shows that when looking at genes that map to the KEGG Cell Cycle pathway, virtually all genes in the pathway scored as essential. By contrast, the number of genes from the same pathway that were found to be essential in the same cell line using an shRNA library were significantly fewer. This makes sense in terms of the way genome-scale knock-down or knock-out screens are performed because these screens rely on cells undergoing several rounds of cell division after infection by the vector library before the sequencing of the bar codes in the constructs that is used to determine the level of gene drop out. So, analysis of the SUM-159 data shows that, when using CRISPR to knock out genes, basically every gene in the Cell Cycle pathway was found to be essential, which was not the case when shRNA vectors were used that only reduced the expression of the cell cycle genes. Thus, when examining gene essentiality data, it is important to keep these differences in mind as it is not uncommon to see genes that score as hits in the CRISPR screens but did not score as hits in the RNAi screen. When this is the case, it's always important to know if the gene that scored in the CRISPR screen is a common essential.

Having determined that gene essentiality data can be used to functionalize genomic data from the SUM breast cancer cell line panel, we decided to expand this type of functional genomic analysis to a larger panel of breast cancer cell lines. In addition, we developed a series of data mining tools that we launched on the SLKBase that allow anyone to perform this type of orthogonal analysis of the data for any breast cancer cell line using simple mouse clicks. For example, the SLKBase contains an *Oncogene Signature* tool that allows users to choose any cell line and determine the candidate oncogenes that are genomically altered and view their gene essentiality data, and thus quickly determine the Oncogene Signature for any cell line. Users can also choose any cell line and any KEGG pathway and see how genes that were found to be essential map onto these KEGG pathways. Thus, for cell lines with KRAS or HRAS mutations, one can view the MAPK KEGG pathway and see quickly how many other genes from that pathway are essential to that cell line. The SLKBase also has Gene Query tools that allow users to enter any gene and determine quickly which if any cell lines over express that gene, or have copy number alterations or point mutations, and to determine if any of those genomic features are associated with essentiality as determined in the screens.

In summary, gene essentiality data can be used to enhance the power of all types of genomic data and provide deep insights into the biology of any cancer cell line. Accordingly, we next decided to use this type of analysis to examine the relationship between genes considered to be important oncogenes in breast cancer and their essentiality in a large panel of breast cancer cell lines. Then, having identified those genes where genomic alterations and essentiality go together, we analyzed the relationship between gene essentiality and drug sensitivity and the result of that analysis will be presented in chapter 7.

CHAPTER 6

THE RELATIONSHIP BETWEEN GENOMIC ALTERATIONS AND GENE ESSENTIALITY IN HUMAN BREAST CANCER CELL LINES

The overarching hypothesis for the analyses that will be described in this chapter is that gene essentiality screens using either CRISPR based, or shRNA-based screening libraries can be used in conjunction with genomic analysis of key breast cancer genes to identify the best druggable targets in breast cancer cells, and by extension in other types of cancer cells as well. As a starting point to address this hypothesis, I analyzed three well known breast cancer genes that have long been validated as effective druggable targets in breast cancer patients to determine how the genomic features associated with these genes are associated with gene essentiality.

The relationship between overexpression of the estrogen receptor gene (ESR1) and gene essentiality in breast cancer cell lines. I started this analysis by examining the most well understood druggable target in breast cancer; the ESR1 gene that codes for estrogen receptor-alpha (ERα). ERα is known to be overexpressed at the mRNA and protein level in approximately two-thirds of breast cancer patients and ERα expression has long been known to be a predictive factor for response to endocrine therapies such as selective estrogen receptor modulators (SERMs) like tamoxifen, selective estrogen receptor degraders (SERDs) like fulvestrant, as well as aromatase inhibitors (AI) like anastrozole. Based on recent work from a number of laboratories, there are data in the public domain that were derived from either CRISPR or shRNA-based essentiality screens that have been carried out with approximately 70 human breast cancer cell lines. In addition, each of these cell lines has been evaluated for copy number and expression of ESR1 and have been characterized for their sensitivity to several anti-estrogen targeted drugs. Thus, I wanted to start by analyzing the relationship between ESR1 gene essentiality and expression at the mRNA level across a panel of breast cancer cell lines.

The left panel of figure 6.1 shows the relationship between essentiality and expression of ESR1 based on the RNAi screen data for approximately 70 breast cancer cell lines. The methods used to quantify the screen data have been published previously. The analysis pipeline yields a CERES score that indicates the degree of essentiality of every gene that was screened. Using this method, a CERES score of -0.5 was determined to be the cut-point for gene essentiality. Thus, any gene in any cell line with a CERES score of -0.5 *or less* is considered a screen hit, or essential in that cell line. Since in ERα positive cells, the ESR1 gene is overexpressed compared to normal cells, we chose to use for this analysis, a log-fold increase in ESR1 levels of 2.0 or greater to indicate overexpression of the gene at the mRNA level.

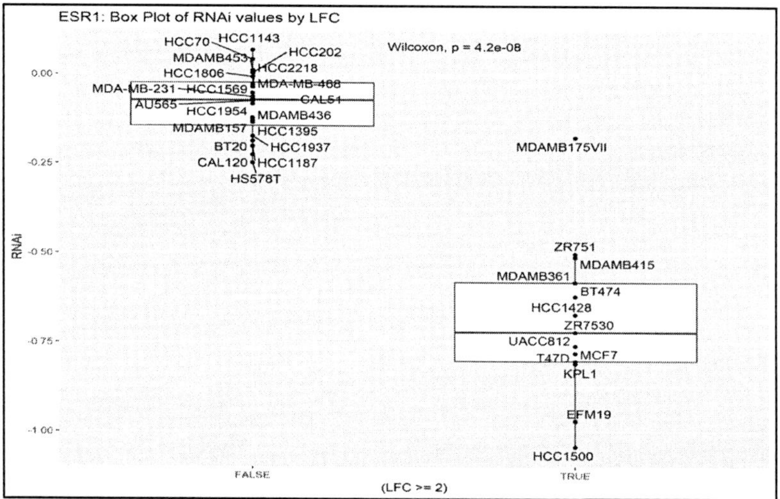

Figure 6.1. Relationship between overexpression of ESR1 and ESR1 gene essentialness. The grouping of cells on the left are considered ER-negative whereas those on the right overexpress ESR1 by at least 2-fold and all of the lines except for 1 have CERES scores ≤ -0.5

The box and whisker plots shown in figure 6.1 shows the ER-positive cell lines on the right and the ER-negative cell lines on the left part of the figure. As can be seen from this figure, for ESR1 there was a clear separation in gene essentiality that was associated with ESR1 expression. This was found using RNAi screens and a similar result was obtained using CRISPR screen data (not shown). As can be seen in the figure, there is a clear and strong association between overexpression of ESR1 and its essentiality as measured in both screens. This analysis yielded Wilcoxon p-values on the order of 10^{-7} to 10^{-8} for the CRISPR and RNAi data respectively. Thus, for the most well characterized genomic feature of breast cancer, ERα overexpression, there is a clear association of the key genomic feature with essentiality of the gene. This is a good start.

The relationship between amplification and overexpression of the ERBB2 gene (HER2) and gene essentiality in breast cancer cell lines. Next, we turned to the ERBB2 (HER2) oncogene as the amplification and overexpression of this gene has long been known to be both a prognostic factor and a predictive factor for response to several ERBB2-targeted drugs. And as is the case for the ESR1 gene, there is a large panel of human breast cancer cell lines that have been analyzed for essentiality of the ERBB2 oncogene as well as it's amplification and overexpression. Figure 6.2 shows the relationship between ERBB2 essentiality and gene amplification across the cell line panel with the CRISPR-derived data on the left and the RNAi-derived data on the right. These results show that there is a statistically significant association between the genomic feature of gene amplification and essentiality with a Wilcoxon p-value of 0.024 for the CRISPR data and of 10^{-5} for the RNAi data. Here, however, the separation of the sets of cell lines is not as clear-cut as was found for the ESR1 data. As has been published previously, the nature of gene amplification events provides some difficulties in the analysis of CRISPR screen data for genes present in amplified regions of the genome (amplicons). Thus, it is interesting

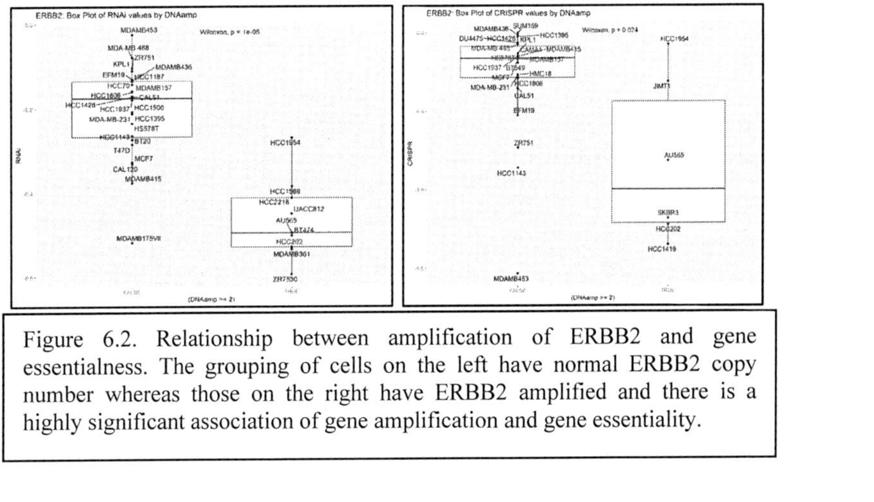

Figure 6.2. Relationship between amplification of ERBB2 and gene essentialness. The grouping of cells on the left have normal ERBB2 copy number whereas those on the right have ERBB2 amplified and there is a highly significant association of gene amplification and gene essentiality.

that the lower p-value associated with the CRISPR screen data can be attributed to the observation that the ERBB2 gene was found to be essential in the CRISPR screen for the ZR751 and HCC1143 cell lines even though the gene is not amplified in these cells. ERBB2 was not found to be essential in these two cell lines in the RNAi screen, suggesting that the CRISPR result for this gene represents a false positive. Results from two other cell lines contribute to the differences observed between the two screening methods. The HCC1954 cell line has a high-level amplification and overexpression of the ERBB2 oncogene and yet the gene was not a hit in either screen. Based on drug sensitivity data that will be described later, this result may represent a false-negative because the cells are highly sensitive to an ERBB2 specific inhibitor, but this remains unclear at this time. The CRISPR data also show that for the JIMT1 cell line, ERBB2 was not essential even though this gene amplified and overexpressed. It is well known that JIMT1 cells are resistant to ERBB2/HER2 targeted drugs (again discussed in more detail in the next section). This suggests that in this cell line, the CRISPR results shows that ERBB2 is not essential in the JIMT1 cell line, even in the setting of gene amplification. The JIMT1 cell line was not analyzed in the RNAi screen, and this further adds to the smaller p-value obtained using the RNAi based data.

These caveats aside, the data still point to a strong association between amplification of ERBB2 and its essentiality in breast cancer cell lines. We also found that for this panel of breast cancer cell lines, there is highly statistically significant correlation between ERBB2 amplification and overexpression (Correlation coefficient = 0.921). This result shows that breast cancer cell lines accurately reflect what is observed in primary tumors and patient samples regarding the relationship between amplification of ERBB2 and its expression at the mRNA and protein levels. Given that the correlation coefficient for amplification and overexpression of ERBB2 in the cell line panel, it is not surprising that the relationship between expression of ERBB2 and gene essentiality observed in the screens mimics that which was observed for gene amplification. Thus, for this second most well studied genomic alteration in breast cancer, the relationship between the key genomic features and essentiality remains strong, but less so than for ESR1.

At this point, a discussion of how gene amplification events result in activation of certain oncogenes in cancer cells is warranted. Unlike the case for ESR1 as described earlier or point mutational events like that for PIK3CA that will be discussed below, both of which only impact the specific gene of interest, gene amplification events occur over discreet genomic regions that always contain multiple genes; sometimes 50 genes or more! It has been known for many years that, within amplicons, only those genes that are overexpressed in the context of gene amplification are considered candidate oncogenes. Typically, even after this filtering method is applied, amplicons always contain more than one, and often several, candidate oncogenes. Within the 17q14 amplified region that results in ERBB2 amplification, there are several other interesting and biologically important genes such as TOPO2 and GRB7 that are likely to play a role in the biology of breast cancer cells with the amplicon. The question that must always be kept in mind is, what is the gene in the amplicon that provides the selective advantage that results in the retention of the amplicon in most or all the cells in the population. It is formally possible that different oncogenes from the same amplicon can be the driver gene in different cell lines and patients and this must always be kept in mind when analyzing screening data or drug sensitivity data with respect to the presence of a discreet amplicon. This is important for interpretation of screen data for oncogenes that are present within amplicons because, whereas ERBB2 is likely to be the driving oncogene in the majority of breast cancers with the ERBB2 amplicon, it is possible that for some cancer cells, a different gene in the region, say GRB7, is the oncogenic driver and is therefore more essential than ERBB2. In such cases, one would *not* predict ERBB2 to score as essential in the screen. Thus, this important aspect of the biology of amplification events in cancer is likely to play a role in the lower p-values observed when analyzing the association between ERBB2 amplification and gene essentiality as compared to the ESR1 data described above. And indeed, this is likely the explanation for why in JIMT1 cells, ERBB2 is not essential, and explains why the cells are

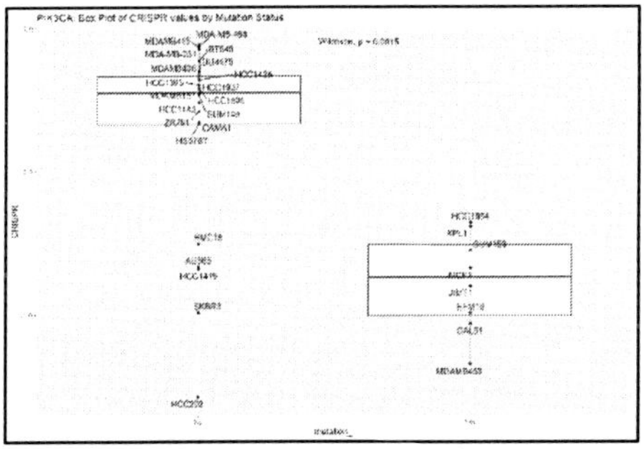

Figure 6.3. Relationship between point mutations in PIK3CA and gene essentialness. The grouping of cells on the left have wild-type PIK3CA copy number whereas those on the right have recurrent PIK3CA mutations. There is a highly significant association between PIK3CA mutations and gene essentiality. Further, PIK3CA is essential in PIK3CA wild-type cell lines that also have an ERBB2 amplification.

resistant to ERBB2 targeted drugs as well. As we will see later, this caveat is of great importance to another candidate breast cancer oncogene, FGFR1, which is found in the 8p11-p12 amplified region that is observed in approximately 15% of breast cancers but is not a driving oncogene.

The relationship between point mutations in the PIK3CA gene and essentiality in breast cancer cell lines. With the advent of deep sequencing capabilities for cancer, many breast cancer specimens and cell lines have been subjected to whole exome sequencing. As a result of these studies the PIK3CA gene, that is central to phosphatidyl inositol 3' kinase (PI3'K) signaling, has been identified as one that is commonly mutated in primary breast cancer and breast cancer cell lines. And as one might expect, there are many breast cancer cell lines that have recurrent mutations in this important oncogene. Therefore, I examined the relationship between point mutations in the PIK3CA oncogene and essentiality of the gene in the panel of breast cancer cell lines. Figure 6.3 shows the results of this analysis. Once again, it is clear that there is a statistically significant association between the presence of point mutations in PIK3CA and essentiality of the gene across the cell line panel. Once again however, there are some interesting discrepancies in the data that contribute to p-values that are higher than what was observed for ESR1. Whereas PIK3CA was found to be essential in every cell line bearing point mutations in the gene, both the CRISPR and RNAi based screens also identified cell lines for which PIK3CA was found to be essential in the *absence* of point mutations. Interestingly, all these PIK3CA wild-type cell lines have amplifications and overexpression of ERBB2! This result suggests that the PIK3CA oncogene is essential in breast cancer cells in *two* genomic contexts: the presence of activating point mutations, and the presence of ERBB2 amplifications. This later finding was unexpected and has interesting implications for how the PI3'kinase pathway is activated when ERBB2 amplifications are present.

Thus, the gene essentiality data indicate the prime importance of the PIK3CA oncogene, as opposed to other members of the PI3'kinase family, in the context of ERBB signaling. As we will see later, this dependency of ERBB2 oncogenic signaling on PIK3CA signaling has an impact on the sensitivity of some breast cancer cells to ERBB2 targeted drugs.

Related to this topic is the finding from deep sequencing studies that even though the ESR1 gene is rarely mutated in primary breast cancer, point mutations in this gene that render the ERα independent of estrogen for signaling has been detected in approximately 30% of metastatic breast cancers (Kuang et al. 2018; Pejerrey et al. 2018; Zhang et al. 2018). Unfortunately, there are no known breast cancer cell lines derived from metastatic lesions with these point mutations so it is not possible here to examine the relationship between ESR1 mutations and essentiality, though one would certainly predict that this gene would be similarly essential in this context.

The relationship between genomic features of other candidate breast cancer genes and essentiality in breast cancer cell lines. The analyses described on the preceding section were focused on genes that are commonly altered in one or more genomic features in a significant subset of breast cancer. Choosing those genes allows for a rigorous statistical analysis of the association between some important genomic feature and gene essentiality. In addition to these more common genomic alterations, there are some breast cancer cell lines that exhibit genomic alterations in genes not commonly found in breast cancer. For example, the DU4475 cell line, which was derived from a dermal metastasis of a patient with breast cancer, is known to have a point mutation in the BRAF oncogene. The V600E mutation is the same one commonly observed in melanoma, and which is associated with sensitivity to the targeted drug Vemurafenib. Examination of the gene essentiality data for this cell line shows that BRAF is highly essential in this cell line, but not in any other breast cancer cell lines (https://sumlineknowledgebase.com/?page_id=3415).

A small number of breast cancer cell lines have point mutations in either the HRAS and KRAS oncogenes, and once again, in these cell lines the mutant RAS oncogenes were found to be essential in the context of those mutations. Finally, the MDA-MB157 cell line has a CCNE1 gene amplification and this gene was a hit in the CRISPR screen (https://sumlineknowledgebase.com/?page_id=3380).

The results presented above help to solidify the argument that gene essentiality can be used to identify the driving oncogenes in breast cancer cell lines, and this is the starting point for further discussions about the relationship between gene essentiality and drug sensitivity. The results presented above notwithstanding, not all our analyses of relationships between potentially important cancer genes and essentiality yielded positive results.

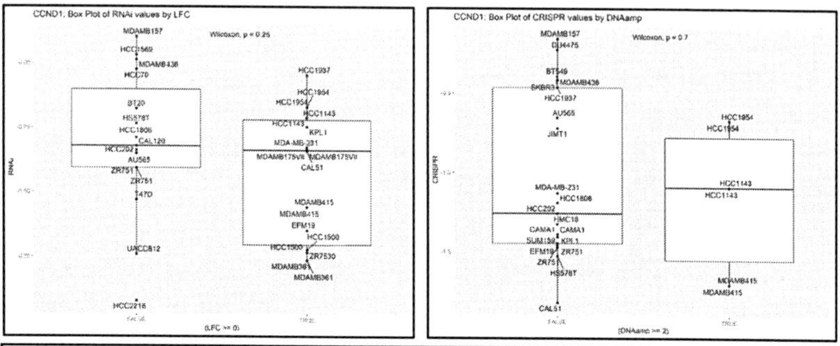

Figure 6.4 Relationship between amplification of CCND1 and gene essentiality in breast cancer cell lines

For example, the CCND1 oncogene, which is located at chromosome 11q14 is part of an amplicon frequently present in breast cancer cells (Hui et al. 1997; Bautista and Theillet 1998; Kwek et al. 2009). Because CCND1 is amplified in the context of a well mapped amplicon, there are other interesting genes in this region, such as GAB2, CTTN, EMSY, and others that have been implicated in breast and other cancers. Thus, examining the relationship between CCND1 amplification and essentiality could shed some light on the importance of this gene in the context of the gene amplification event at 14q14.

The box and whisker plots below shown in Figure 6.4 demonstrates quite clearly that, unlike for ERBB2, there is no association between CCND1 gene amplification and gene essentiality determined using either the CRISPR or the RNAi screen data. That is not to say that CCND1 is not an essential gene in some breast cancer cell lines; it clearly is as indicated by the number of cell lines with CERES scores for CCND1 that are significantly less than -0.5. What the data indicate, however, is that for CCND1, essentiality is *independent* of the gene amplification event.

In a similar vein, I performed an analysis to examine the relationship between overexpression of the epidermal growth factor receptor (EGFR) gene and gene essentiality in breast cancer cell lines. It has long been known that EGFR overexpression is common in ER-negative breast cancer, and indeed, EGFR expression is inversely correlated with ER-expression (Suo et al. 2002). For that reason, there was once excitement in

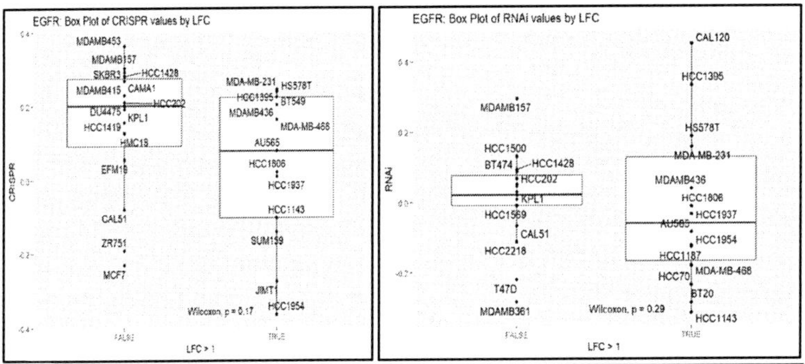

Figure 6.5 Relationship between expression of EGFR and gene essentiality in breast cancer cell lines.

the field about EGFR as a drug target in ER-negative breast cancer. Unfortunately, clinical trials of drugs such as gefitinib and erlotinib in breast cancer did not indicate any clinical benefit associated with targeting EGFR when overexpressed (Agrawal et al. 2005). The box and whisker plots in figure 6.5 show that this is indeed what would have been predicted had gene essentiality data been available to address this question. These results show that EGFR was almost never found to be essential in breast cancer cell lines regardless of the level of overexpression, and indeed, there was no correlation between expression level and essentialness. Even for cell lines like MDA-MB-468 and BT20 in which EGFR is both amplified and highly overexpressed, EGFR did not come close to scoring as essential in either the CRISPR or RNAi screens. Thus, once again, the lack of an association between a specific genomic feature and gene essentiality is consistent with clinical findings using specific targeted drugs.

This distinction is important because, as we will see, we hypothesize that when it comes to driving oncogenes in cancer cells only those that are essential are good drug targets. In the best cases, an effective and specific targeted drug will have the same effect on cells as the knock-down or knock out of the gene. By contrast, if gene knock-down or knock-out failed to have a significant effect on the cancer cells in which they are genomically altered, then it's unlikely, and perhaps impossible for a drug to the same target to be effective in affecting the proliferation or survival of the breast cancer cells. The data above are consistent with this notion as the products of the ESR1, ERBB2 and mutant PIK3CA genes have proven themselves to be excellent drug targets, whereas CCND1 and EGFR have not.

In summary, our analyses of several genes and oncogenes thought to be important in breast cancer serve to highlight those genes for which specific genomic features are associated with, or not associated with, gene essentiality. Furthermore, based on current clinical evidence, we can see that only the genes for which essentiality tracks with the genomic feature are the genes known to be good drug targets. By contrast, for those genes where the genomic feature is not associated with essentiality, the clinical data are consistent and have shown these genes not to be good drug targets.

The relationship between amplification and overexpression of FGFR genes and essentiality in breast cancer cell lines. The role of the family of FGFR genes in breast cancer is worthy of a separate discussion now that we've analyzed other important breast cancer genes in terms of essentiality. Because the FGFR genes code for receptor tyrosine kinases, much like ERBB2 and EGFR, and because they are amplified and overexpressed in breast cancer with some frequency, this gene family has been the subject of intensive investigation in both the laboratory and the clinic, and as we will see, the studies and results obtained are not without controversy. So, the question arises; can an analysis of the relationship between amplification of FGFR family members and gene essentiality help to shed light on this controversy?

Based on the results of the analysis of the five genes that are considered to be important in breast cancer biology, combined with our previous published results, we conclude that gene essentiality is an excellent indicator of dominant driving oncogenic activity of candidate oncogenes. Conversely, lack of association between genomic alterations in candidate oncogenes with gene essentiality suggests that the genomic alterations in these genes are only *correlated* with the biology of breast cancer, and do not play an important *functional* role in either the proliferation or the survival of cancer cells bearing the oncogenic feature.

Several years ago, after developing the panel of SUM breast cancer cell lines and finding that only two of them (the expected ratio) had an amplification of the ERBB2 oncogene, we set out to discover and characterize the driving oncogenic events in the other members of the cell line panel. We were fortunate at that time to be collaborating with Jeffry Trent's group at the National Human Genome Research Institute (NHGRI), and a member of that group, Dr. Ollie O.P. Kallioniemi was working to develop chromosome comparative genomic hybridization (CGH) technology as well as some of the first cDNA gene expression arrays for breast cancer. In collaboration with the Kallioniemi lab, we examined the SUM breast cancer cell line panel for regions of focal gene amplification and for expression of the 500 genes that were present on these early-generation arrays (Forozan et al. 1999). From this work, we confirmed that the SUM-190 and SUM-225 cell lines had focal regions of gene amplification in the 17q14 region, the location of the ERBB2 oncogene, and we also discovered that three of the SUM lines harbored focal regions of gene amplification in the 8p11.p12 genomic region. This was an interesting and surprising discovery because while this region of the genome was already known to be amplified in 10 to 15% of breast cancers, there were no other cell lines in which this region was known to be amplified. Thus, the SUM-44, SUM-52, and SUM-225 cell lines presented a novel opportunity to study this genomic region more thoroughly. What made the observations from the chromosome CGH even more compelling was the observations made using the expression arrays (which fortunately contained cDNAs for FGFR1and 2) which showed that while FGFR1 was expressed at the mRNA level in SUM-44 cells, it was not expressed in either SUM-52 or SUM-225 cells (Forozan et al. 2000; Kononen et al. 2001). The suggestion from these observations was that, while it was possible that FGFR1 was the driving oncogene in SUM-44 cells, it could not be so in the other two cell lines since the gene was not expressed. Thus, we reasoned, there must be other driving oncogenes from this genomic region to be identified and characterized for their transforming activity and, later, for their essentialness. Adding to the compelling nature of this story was the finding that SUM-52 cells also harbored a focal amplification in the 10q26 region, which is the genomic location of the FGFR2 oncogene, and the cDNA array data showed that this gene was 40-fold overexpressed at the mRNA level, whereas FGFR1 was not expressed at detectable levels in these cells.

It is important to note that at the time that we and others were exploring this region of the genome, there were only two known candidate oncogenes in the 8p11 amplicon. FGFR1 had long been known to reside in this region and was thus widely considered (without direct evidence) to be the driving oncogene. Interestingly, the Pierre Chambon laboratory in France proposed that another gene in the region, then known as NSD3, as the dominant driver of amplification in the region (Angrand et al. 2001).

Given the widely held assumption that FGFR1 was the driving oncogene from the 8p11 region, coupled with our finding that SUM-44 cells harbored an FGFR1 amplification that was associated with FGFR1 expression at the mRNA level, we sought to investigate the role of this candidate oncogene in the growth potential of SUM-44 cells. We performed experiments to measure FGFR1 expression at the protein level and we were surprised to find that FGFR1 protein was not detectable in these cells by western blot analysis. We next measured protein expression of FGFR2 in SUM-52 cells. As we published in several subsequent papers, we able to demonstrate high level overexpression of FGFR2 protein in SUM-52 cells, and indeed went on to demonstrate the presence of multiple splice isoforms of the gene that were expressed in these cells, some of which were potently transforming (Tannheimer, Rehemtulla, and Ethier 2000; Kononen et al. 2001; Moffa, Tannheimer, and Ethier 2004; Moffa and Ethier 2007). Next, we performed experiments to examine the ability of the newly developed drug PD173074 to influence the growth of the cell lines with the 8p11 amplifications. Fortunately for these experiments, PD173074 had been shown to be a pan-specific inhibitor of the FGFR family, and thus equally effective at inhibiting FGFR1 and FGFR2. Not surprisingly, we found SUM-52 cells to be exquisitely sensitive to PD173074 and this was later demonstrated by other labs as well. This is critical to the story of FGFR1 because, as one would predict from our inability to measure FGFR1 protein expression in SUM-44 cells, these cells were unresponsive to PD173074. In later work, we discovered that another SUM cell line, SUM-185, harbors an amplification and overexpression of FGFR3, and these cells too are exquisitely sensitive to PD173074.

These results indicate that despite the amplification of FGFR1 and its expression at the mRNA level in SUM-44 cells, the gene does not play a role in the proliferative potential of these cells in vitro. Thus, we argued that FGFR1 is not a driving oncogene in any of the three cell lines that we developed that harbor the 8p11.p12 region of gene amplification (Ray et al. 2004; Yang, Albertson, and Ethier 2004).

The work carried out to that point, provided positive evidence for a transforming function and driving oncogenic function for FGFR2 in SUM-52 cells and FGFR3 in SUM-185 cells. By contrast, all the evidence that we had for FGFR1 was negative, and negative data are difficult to interpret. Thus, it remained possible that FGFR1 amplification could influence proliferation and/or survival of breast cancer cells *in vivo* in a way that was not easily detectable *in vitro*.

As described earlier, my laboratory performed genome-scale RNAi based essentiality screens on the entire panel of SUM breast cancer cell lines. The complete results of these experiments can be found on the SLKBase, but relevant to the present discussion, we found that FGFR2 is highly essential in SUM-52 cells and FGFR3 is highly essential in SUM-185 cells (Guest et al. 2016). By contrast, we have never identified FGFR1 as an essential gene in any of our cell lines, including those with the 8p11-p12 amplified region.

To examine this question further, we looked at additional breast cancer cell lines with FGFR1 gene amplifications and overexpression to determine if FGFR1 is essential in any of these cell lines (data available on the SLKBase). Once again, analysis of the breast cancer cell line data in our database did not reveal FGFR1 to be essential in any of the 70 breast cancer cell lines regardless of amplification status of the gene.

As will be discussed in a subsequent chapter, it is also possible to use drug sensitivity data to identify essential genes in breast cancer. Therefore, we took this alternate approach to investigate further the possibility that FGFR1 is a good drug target, despite the gene essentiality data. Beyond the SUM lines described above, there are two breast cancer cell lines with high level amplification of FGFR1 (MDA-MB134VI and CAL120) and six cell lines with lower levels of FGFR1 amplification (JIMT1, CAMA1, HCC1599, ZR751, MDA-MB157, UACC812). Some, but not all of these lines, exhibit FGFR1 expression at the mRNA level. While there are no drug sensitivity data available for the MDA-MB134VI cells, none of the other breast cancer cell lines described above exhibit sensitivity to PD173074. Taking the converse approach, when looking at the several hundred cell lines present in the Genomics of Drug Sensitivity in Cancer database to identify the cells most sensitive to PD173074, only two breast cancer cell lines show even moderate sensitivity, and neither of them exhibit FGFR1 gene amplification. Thus, FGFR1, like CCND1 and EGFR, is not predicted to be a good drug target based on gene essentiality, and this result holds up at the level of targeted drug sensitivity.

Despite the volume and scope of negative data on FGFR1 as a driving oncogene in breast cancer, several clinical trials have been carried out using some of the newest generation of FGFR-targeted drugs. And as was the case for EGFR overexpression described earlier, these clinical studies also have not identified any clinical benefit associated with these targeted drugs in patients with FGFR1 amplification and overexpression (Andre et al. 2013; Brady et al. 2013; De Luca et al. 2017; Perez-Garcia et al. 2018).

Thus, for the FGFR family of oncogenes, we have demonstrated a relationship between amplification/overexpression of FGFR2 and FGFR3 in a small panel of breast cancer cell lines, and indeed in these cells, essentiality is associated with exquisite drug sensitivity. By contrast, there is still no evidence that, in the context of the 8p11 amplicon, FGFR1 is a driving oncogene that would be associated with sensitivity to an FGFR targeted drug.

Given those findings, we wanted to determine if there are other oncogenes within the 8p11 region that have scored as hits in essentiality screens in breast cancer cell lines. The answer to that question is a rather surprising yes. In our cell line panel, the histone acetylase gene KAT6A scored as a hit in the screen of SUM-52 cells. In work subsequent to this discovery, we validated the transforming function of KAT6A. This gene also scored as a hit in the project Achilles based CRISPR screen of ZR75-1 cells, which also harbors the 8p11 amplicon. Subsequent to these findings, other evidence was reported in the literature on the potential importance of KAT6A as on oncogene and possible implications of that genomic event for drug sensitivity (Turner-Ivey et al. 2014).

The relationship between transforming function and essentiality for breast cancer oncogenes. There is another interesting and possibly surprising finding that has emerged from our analysis of the relationship between genomic alterations and essentiality. That concerns the relationship, or lack thereof, between the transforming function of an oncogene and its essentiality in established cancer cells. As mentioned earlier, my laboratory spent many years studying the candidate oncogenes present in the 8p11 amplicon found in about 15% of breast cancers. To perform our experiments, we took the same approach that we had used previously to document and understand the transforming function of the ERBB2 oncogene. These approaches involved testing the ability of candidate oncogene overexpression to induce growth factor independence, anchorage independence, motility, invasive capacity, etc. when overexpressed in immortalized but otherwise normal human mammary epithelial cells. In performing these experiments, we identified several genes in the 8p11 amplicon that, when overexpressed, could "transform" MCF-10A cells to one or more of these altered phenotypes (Yang et al. 2006; Streicher et al. 2007; Yang et al. 2009; Yang et al. 2010; G. Wang et al. 2012; Turner-Ivey et al. 2014; Irish et al. 2016; Turner-Ivey et al. 2017; Rutkovsky et al. 2019). From our work, the most potently transforming gene from the amplicon was WHSC1L1, now and previously known as NSD3 (recall the Pierre Chambon prediction from 2001). And yet, we never did identify

NSD3 as an essential gene in our cell lines with the 8p11 amplicon, nor did the gene hit in any of the RNAi or CRISPR screens performed in Project Achilles. Subsequently, we used our database to look at relationships between other known or suspected transforming oncogenes and essentiality and identified several other genes that did not score in the screens. Thus, these observations suggest the rather intriguing idea that not all transforming oncogenes are essential to the proliferation and survival of established cancer cells. If that is the case, as we suggested earlier, the presence of an oncogene in the oncogene signature of a cancer cell line or specimen is not enough to predict its value as a drug target.

In summary, our findings indicate that gene essentiality is an excellent way to identify genes that are most likely to be good targets in cancer cells with specific genomic or expression alterations associated with the genes. Thus, we conclude that gene essentiality is necessary for a gene to be a good target for novel drugs in breast cancer. The next question is, is gene essentiality sufficient to predict targeted drug sensitivity?

CHAPTER 7

THE RELATIONSHIP BETWEEN GENE ESSENTIALITY AND DRUG SENSITIVITY IN HUMAN BREAST CANCER CELL LINES

The results of the analyses presented in Chapter 6 strongly suggests that gene essentiality is one way to identify oncogenes that could be good drug targets. So, if gene essentiality is an important predictor of targeted drug sensitivity, is it sufficient? That is, are all cell lines that have genomic alterations in essential genes that are also druggable, sensitive to the cognate targeted drugs? In a perfect world, a good drug against an essential target should act just like an shRNA or an sgRNA against the same target. That is, in a perfect world, the drugs and targeting vectors should be equally efficacious, given the essentiality of the target. To address this question, we next focused our attention on those oncogenes found to be essential in breast cancer cell lines and examined how these cell lines respond to several targeted drugs.

Before going on to describe the results of this analysis, I want to provide the conclusion first. Because in knowing the conclusion, one can examine the results and the various caveats associated with them in a better light. The conclusion is this: In every case that I have examined, the cell lines with the highest levels of sensitivity to oncogene targeted drugs are those in which the target gene is genomically altered and was found to be essential in one or both essentiality screens. That is the good news. The not-so-good news is that the overall correlation coefficient between gene essentiality and targeted drug sensitivity is rarely greater that approximately 0.5 and this is because there are always cell lines in which the target gene is genomically altered, was found to be essential in the cell line, and yet the cells are not highly sensitive to the drug. This too is *always* the case. And thus, the overall conclusion is that, whereas gene essentiality and genomic alterations are *correlated* with targeted drug sensitivity, the presence of a genomic alteration in what is known as a good target gene is not sufficient to predict sensitivity to the targeted drug(s) with high confidence. This is important because we know for certain that this same problem occurs in the clinic. There are many targeted drugs associated with genomic features that are used as predictive biomarkers that result in patients being treated with cognate targeted drugs. But only a fraction of the patients have good responses to the drugs. Indeed, we have long known that only about one-quarter of patients with HER2 amplified breast cancers respond to Trastuzumab, and the same has been observed for other oncogene targeted drugs. Thus, the ultimate challenge, and the one that we want to address in this work, is how to predict which patients will be sensitive or resistant to targeted drugs given the genomic features of the individual specimen. And for those patients with a specific targetable genomic alteration that are not sensitive to the targeted drug, can we predict which other drugs that they might be sensitive to? If we can accomplish this, or even make significant progress towards this goal, this will move us closer to our goal of adding precision to the development of targeted drug treatment plans for patients.

Before we delve into these data further, it's important to set the stage and describe how drug sensitivity data are reported in the GDSC database. Drug sensitivity data for cancer cell lines were derived by determining the IC50 doses for hundreds of targeted drugs across hundreds of cancer cell lines. Details of how the analyses were conducted are available on the GDSC website (https://www.cancerrxgene.org/). Based on those extensive measurements, drug sensitivity data are reported on the GDSC website in two ways. First, when looking at data for individual drugs, the IC50 values for that drug in μM are shown for all the cell lines that were tested with the drug and are presented as a rank-ordered list of cell lines based on sensitivity. Cells that are most sensitive to the drug in question have the lowest IC50s whereas cells that are most resistant have the highest IC50s. The dynamic range of these data are particularly noteworthy as for some drugs, IC50 values can range over 1000 to 10,000-fold demonstrating the tremendous range in sensitivity of cancer cell lines to individual targeted drugs! These observations demonstrate the importance of properly identifying cell lines, specimens, and patients with the highest sensitivity to specific targeted drugs and to avoid treating patients with drugs to which they are intrinsically resistant. Such treatments provide no clinical benefit but come with all the side-effects/toxicities. Thus, by using these drug sensitivity data, one can quickly determine the cells that are most and least sensitive to any drug in the database.

Alternatively, one can examine the relative sensitivity of all drugs in any particular cell line. For this type of analysis, drug sensitivity data are presented as Z-scores. Each Z-score unit represents one standard deviation from the geometric mean of IC50s for a given drug across all cell lines. Thus, for each cell line in the database, the drugs to which the cells are most sensitive have the lowest Z-scores and cells that are most resistant have the highest Z-scores. Thus, Z-scores range from approximately -4.0 to +4.0. Drugs that are most effective in a given cell line have negative Z-scores, whereas drugs to which cells are resistant have strong positive Z-scores. A Z-score of 0 indicates that the cells have average sensitivity to the drug in question.

For the analyses to be presented here, we will use Z-scores as our measure of drug sensitivity. This is most convenient because a particular Z-score, say -2.0, has the same biological meaning for any drug in any cell line. By contrast, because intrinsic drug potencies of individual drugs are so highly variable, an IC50 of 1.0 μM might indicate high sensitivity for one drug, but low sensitivity for another more potent or active drug. Z-scores, on the other hand, have the same meaning for all drugs in all cell lines. Within the GDSC database, cells are considered highly sensitive to individual drugs when the Z-score for the drug is -1.5 or less.

ESR1 gene essentiality and targeted drug sensitivity. As in the previous chapter, we begin this analysis by looking at the sensitivity of ER-positive breast cancer cell lines to a series of clinically useful ER targeted drugs. Recall from Chapter 6 that the ESR1 gene was found to be essential in all the ER+ breast cancer cell lines. Thus, this is again, a great starting point for the analysis. As in the previous chapter, the gene essentiality data we are using come from Project Achilles and the drug sensitivity data come from the Genomics of Drug Sensitivity in Cancer Database (GDSC).

Let's now turn to the question of how sensitivity to drugs that target the estrogen receptor are related to the essentiality of the ESR1 gene in ER-positive breast cancer cell lines. At the present time, there are several different drugs used to treat patients with ER-positive breast cancer. Tamoxifen (TAM) is the drug that has been in use the longest and there is rich clinical data on the efficacy of this drug in patients. Tamoxifen is the gold-standard for the type of drug known as Selective Estrogen Receptor Modulators (SERMs). Tamoxifen acts by binding to the estrogen receptor and in that way prevents the natural ligand, 17-β-estradiol, from binding and activating the receptor. Interestingly, Tamoxifen is an estrogen antagonist in breast cancer cells but is a partial agonist of the estrogen receptor in other tissues. For this reason, Tamoxifen is an effective inhibitor of estrogen action in breast cancer cells but acts more like an

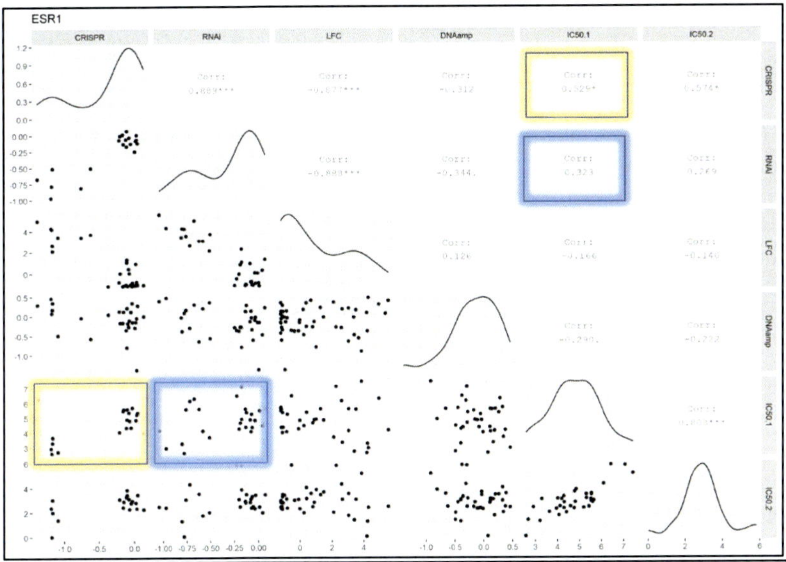

Figure 7.1 Correlation plots for genomic and gene essentiality data for ESR1 in the breast cancer cell line panel. Yellow highlighted box shows the data for the association of CRISPR based essentiality and the IC50 for GDC0810. Blue highlighted boxes show values based on RNAi screen data.

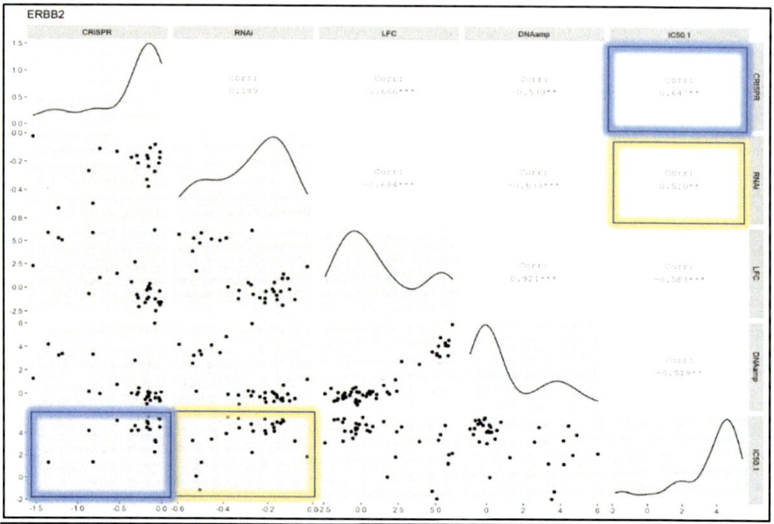

Figure 7.2 Correlation plots for genomic and gene essentiality data for ERBB2 in the breast cancer cell line panel. Blue highlighted box shows the data for the association of CRISPR based essentiality and the IC50 for CP724714. Yellow highlighted boxes show values based on RNAi screen data.

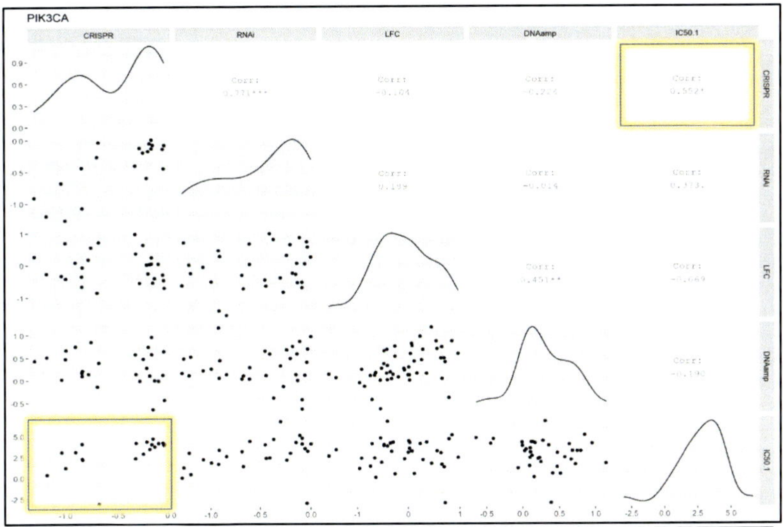

Figure 7.3 Correlation plots for genomic and gene essentiality data for PIK3CA in the breast cancer cell line panel. Yellow highlighted box shows the data for the association of CRISPR based essentiality and the IC50 for Alpelisib.

Variant	Cell.line	CRISPR	RNAi	LFC	DNAamp	Z.score.2
ESR1	**MCF7**	**-1.18036952**	**-0.78112115**	**4.193281236**	**0.072386**	**-2.656779**
ESR1	**CAMA1**	**-1.09084778**		**3.407229827**	**-0.495**	**-2.54482**
ESR1	**EFM19**	**-1.18895946**	**-0.97085516**	**4.292021817**	**0.4591**	**-2.291865**
ESR1	**T47D**		**-0.80228517**	**4.23392322**	**-0.3971**	**-1.967374**
ESR1	**HCC1419**	**-1.17260532**		**2.653920144**	**0.1656**	**-1.884934**
ESR1	**MDAMB415**	**-1.16942107**	**-0.51293873**	**2.102237023**	**0.340575**	**-1.503542**
ESR1	DU4475	0.1362821		-1.099977516	-0.0116	-1.15571
ESR1	AU565	-0.20966055	-0.07515477	-0.832497205	0.1178	-1.08924
ESR1	MDAMB361		-0.58339533	3.039952745	0.1876	-1.028283
ESR1	HCC1500		-1.04369729	5.541605976	0.376	-0.975961
ESR1	MDA-MB-231	-0.1135913	-0.06349525	-1.086680693	-0.3614	-0.785143
ESR1	CAL148			-1.168364491	-0.0825	-0.771152
ESR1	MDAMB157	-0.04612554	-0.12993241	-1.060449152	0.1073	-0.761996
ESR1	CAL851			-0.331303062	-0.3993	-0.670034
ESR1	HCC70		0.041941437	0.258877148	-0.49	-0.647553
ESR1	BT20		-0.18799998	0.79977101	-0.2868	-0.444105
ESR1	HCC1806	-0.19423238	-0.00708035	-0.009374967	-0.176	-0.323748
ESR1	MDA-MB-468	-0.06729578	-0.03570804	0.003115977	-0.1125	-0.26525
ESR1	EFM192A			1.493863136	-0.0379	-0.244697
ESR1	HCC1954	0.024217207	-0.083482	0.893327831	-0.1519	-0.220263
ESR1	HCC1937	-0.10260697	-0.1743028	1.024718231	-0.8104	-0.18249
ESR1	HS578T	0.012036171	-0.24852979	-1.140619501	-0.297437	0.112852
ESR1	CAL51	0.036525054	-0.07110116	-0.799582583	-0.0546	0.192077
ESR1	HDQP1			0.216597344	0.1552	0.220394
ESR1	MDAMB436	0.049717758	-0.12321358	-1.086680693	0.261927	0.322114
ESR1	JIMT1	-0.07650913		0.41659801	-0.276511	0.326364
ESR1	MDAMB453	-0.15852926	0.010744388	-1.196653536	-0.1724	0.458215
ESR1	UACC812		-0.76033225	3.512003568	0.1425	0.548188
ESR1	HCC1395	-0.14797668	-0.13559383	-1.168364491	0.112643	0.563096
ESR1	HCC1143	-0.10144188	0.06837317	1.289793225	0.201385	0.574479
ESR1	BT474		-0.62224052	3.050521987	-0.6621	0.575973
ESR1	HCC2157			-1.196653536	-0.4491	0.636943
ESR1	BT549	-0.02716235		-1.196653536	0.3285	0.695894
ESR1	ZR7530		-0.72129899	2.601489172	-0.3102	1.168363
ESR1	HCC1428	-1.38724254	-0.67275976	4.95450119	0.2831	1.341568
ESR1	CAL120		-0.22626741	-0.52394814	-0.3784	1.544801
ESR1	MDAMB175VII		-0.17796122	2.260178632	-0.2938	2.237782
ESR1	BT483			3.867515617	-0.9192	2.624753

Table 7.1. Relationship between ESR1 expression, essentiality, and sensitivity to GDC0810.

Variant	Cell.line	CRISPR	RNAi	LFC	DNAamp	Z.score.1
ESR1	**T47D**		**-0.802285175**	**4.23392322**	**-0.3971**	**-3.341002**
ESR1	**MCF7**	**-1.18036952**	**-0.781121154**	**4.193281236**	**0.072386**	**-2.217613**
ESR1	**MDAMB361**		**-0.583395334**	**3.039952745**	**0.1876**	**-1.491907**
ESR1	HCC1569		-0.052670392	-1.140619501	-0.6261	-0.976834
ESR1	HCC1428	-1.387242538	-0.672759758	4.95450119	0.2831	-0.921562
ESR1	HCC1954	0.024217207	-0.083482001	0.893327831	-0.1519	-0.892774
ESR1	JIMT1	-0.07650913		0.41659801	-0.276511	-0.86876
ESR1	BT549	-0.02716235		-1.196653536	0.3285	-0.867285
ESR1	HCC1500		-1.043697285	5.541605976	0.376	-0.620545
ESR1	DU4475	0.1362821		-1.099977516	-0.0116	-0.602773
ESR1	EFM19	-1.188959455	-0.970855159	4.292021817	0.4591	-0.579059
ESR1	EFM192A			1.493863136	-0.0379	-0.429355
ESR1	CAL120		-0.226267409	-0.52394814	-0.3784	-0.26218
ESR1	MDAMB415	-1.169421071	-0.512938733	2.102237023	0.340575	-0.07861
ESR1	MDA-MB-468	-0.06729578	-0.035708038	0.003115977	-0.1125	-0.036375
ESR1	HCC1806	-0.194232383	-0.007080352	-0.009374967	-0.176	-0.013609
ESR1	UACC812		-0.760332253	3.512003568	0.1425	0
ESR1	HCC1599			0.402522824	0.3249	0
ESR1	CAL148			-1.168364491	-0.0825	0
ESR1	MDA-MB-231	-0.113591305	-0.063495253	-1.086680693	-0.3614	0.029244
ESR1	CAL51	0.036525054	-0.071101155	-0.799582583	-0.0546	0.053098
ESR1	HCC2157			-1.196653536	-0.4491	0.292693
ESR1	AU565	-0.209660546	-0.075154772	-0.832497205	0.1178	0.413629
ESR1	MDAMB453	-0.158529259	0.010744388	-1.196653536	-0.1724	0.425666
ESR1	MDAMB157	-0.046125536	-0.129932413	-1.060449152	0.1073	0.462591
ESR1	HCC70		0.041941437	0.258877148	-0.49	0.470361
ESR1	HS578T	0.012036171	-0.248529787	-1.140619501	-0.297437	0.525394
ESR1	HDQP1			0.216597344	0.1552	0.644026
ESR1	BT474		-0.62224052	3.050521987	-0.6621	0.695099
ESR1	HCC2218		-0.029199221	-0.972221969	-0.0352	0.716685
ESR1	MDAMB175VII		-0.177961216	2.260178632	-0.2938	0.799203
ESR1	HCC1937	-0.102606973	-0.174302805	1.024718231	-0.8104	0.809213
ESR1	CAMA1	-1.090847779		3.407229827	-0.495	0.818577
ESR1	BT20		-0.187999981	0.79977101	-0.2868	0.820859
ESR1	UACC893			0.695881767	0.387	0.873568
ESR1	HCC1143	-0.101441881	0.06837317	1.289793225	0.201385	0.880904
ESR1	HCC1395	-0.14797668	-0.13559383	-1.168364491	0.112643	0.999166
ESR1	CAL851			-0.331303062	-0.3993	1.042064
ESR1	MDAMB436	0.049717758	-0.123213582	-1.086680693	0.261927	1.156737
ESR1	HCC202	0.035574128	0.003893899	-0.924127681	-1.3869	1.199007
ESR1	HCC1419	-1.17260532		2.653920144	0.1656	1.200606
ESR1	BT483			3.867515617	-0.9192	1.994687
ESR1	ZR7530		-0.721298992	2.601489172	-0.3102	2.20956

Table 7.2. Relationship between ESR1 expression, essentiality and sensitivity to Tamoxifen.

Variant	Cell.line	CRISPR	RNAi	LFC	DNAamp	CP724714 Z.score.1
ERBB2	HCC2218		-0.412879752	5.085926364	3.5235	-6.512228
ERBB2	BT474		-0.502029224	4.779979821	3.6675	-5.77877
ERBB2	MDAMB175VII		-0.518655663	1.761804294	0.1792	-4.419212
ERBB2	HCC1419	-1.351421217		5.858527326	4.189	-3.134253
ERBB2	AU565	-0.81489376	-0.495464868	5.854488474	3.3439	-3.095289
ERBB2	MDAMB453	-1.532579796	-0.02423158	2.298230297	1.2681	-2.496664
ERBB2	UACC893			5.899999137	4.6712	-2.238272
ERBB2	DU4475	-0.067051706		-2.433913475	0.019	-1.152206
ERBB2	MDA-MB-468	-0.074025951	-0.079703187	-1.209469731	-0.401	-0.989809
ERBB2	MDAMB361		-0.53421204	3.902117358	2.5961	-0.975548
ERBB2	UACC812		-0.450607423	5.198256237	4.157	-0.858793
ERBB2	CAL851			-0.543207128	0.4595	-0.698149
ERBB2	T47D		-0.286292745	0.560507581	0.2314	-0.325788
ERBB2	HCC1569		-0.384407802	5.340965441	4.8823	-0.292592
ERBB2	HCC1500		-0.207972579	-0.350852711	-0.7226	-0.282167
ERBB2	BT483			2.395847157	0.2715	-0.046626
ERBB2	CAL51	-0.355719982	-0.17093707	0.589073198	0.011	-0.045458
ERBB2	HCC1143	-0.861855521	-0.265565434	-0.66525464	0.170255	-0.044249
ERBB2	MDA-MB-231	-0.275042626	-0.211965409	-1.101676281	0.0894	-0.005125
ERBB2	CAMA1	-0.136003506		0.422877832	0.0638	0.076692
ERBB2	CAL148			1.90295311	0.0148	0.105305
ERBB2	HCC1806	-0.290720436	-0.160191357	-0.761600839	-0.1056	0.119524
ERBB2	HCC1599			-0.355948778	0.5691	0.125323
ERBB2	MCF7	-0.173258166	-0.327824944	-0.257298256	-0.910342	0.267239
ERBB2	HCC1428	-0.019959028	-0.172509257	-0.366880926	-0.6603	0.302553
ERBB2	JIMT1	-0.312425716		2.716116958	2.836604	0.434577
ERBB2	HCC2157			0.770871978	0.2242	0.446333
ERBB2	EFM192A			5.663982249	4.4367	0.592146
ERBB2	BT20		-0.273881933	0.352766186	-0.1969	0.624186
ERBB2	HCC1937	-0.157328692	-0.179569153	-0.127007571	0.1457	0.649099
ERBB2	HCC70		-0.142963938	-0.338695097	-0.4678	0.732642
ERBB2	MDAMB157	-0.168953956	-0.158549776	-1.234905994	-0.3311	0.836555
ERBB2	HS578T	-0.153392581	-0.235331815	-1.032591969	-0.250199	0.884508
ERBB2	EFM19	-0.52682133	-0.130309925	1.501245704	0.779	0.924221
ERBB2	HDQP1			-0.277462708	0.1876	0.962215
ERBB2	MDAMB436	-0.017020248	-0.134415941	-1.807404529	-0.619644	1.092154
ERBB2	HCC1395	-0.028151107	-0.212396361	-1.557616673	-0.415505	1.115574
ERBB2	CAL120		-0.330800845	-1.144537495	-0.1319	1.17848
ERBB2	MDAMB415	-0.152707648	-0.376779018	0.116879292	-0.076872	1.327014

Table 7.3. Relationship between ERBB2 amplification, expression, essentiality and sensitivity to CP724714.

Variant	Cell.line	CRISPR	RNAi	LFC	DNAamp	Z.score.2	mutation
PIK3CA	**MDAMB361**		**-1.284109778**	**-0.64251067**	**0.1533**	**-2.538572**	**p.E545K, p.K567R**
PIK3CA	**MDAMB453**	**-1.17563853**	**-1.197997**	**-0.262086925**	**0.5131**	**-2.263952**	**p.H1047R**
PIK3CA	**UACC893**			**0.114218179**	**0.4061**	**-2.243956**	**p.H1047R**
PIK3CA	**CAL148**			**-0.958749693**	**-0.0654**	**-1.794044**	**p.D350N, p.H1047R**
PIK3CA	**BT20**		**-0.604229288**	**0.652638094**	**0.0202**	**-1.735854**	**p.P539R, p.H1047R**
PIK3CA	**EFM19**	**-0.996488226**	**-1.267484115**	**0.69426519**	**0.4686**	**-1.680552**	**p.H1047L**
PIK3CA	**HCC1954**	**-0.680242059**	**-0.038079112**	**0.713827456**	**0.3852**	**-1.472164**	**p.H1047R**
PIK3CA	HCC1599			0.645864866	0.72	-1.471779	
PIK3CA	T47D		-0.922765214	0.447875567	1.1486	-1.378822	p.H1047R
PIK3CA	BT474		-0.994225686	-0.525121331	0.2456	-1.277687	p.K111N
PIK3CA	MDAMB175VII		-0.666812199	-0.745604162	0.0907	-1.172911	
PIK3CA	HCC1569		-0.238750895	0.283052296	0.6627	-1.067204	
PIK3CA	AU565	-0.835473383	-1.075803484	-0.07422691	0.21	-0.987725	
PIK3CA	EFM192A			-0.91803602	0.2292	-0.918925	p.C420R
PIK3CA	MCF7	-0.840496119	-0.440093034	-0.663389399	0.095766	-0.914938	p.E545K
PIK3CA	HS578T	-0.334097503	-0.405952836	0.967113885	0.572631	-0.867087	
PIK3CA	UACC812		-0.841867499	-1.557977159	0.1227	-0.736091	
PIK3CA	HDQP1			-0.089687014	0.2403	-0.531603	
PIK3CA	HCC1143	-0.260664369	-0.20236643	0.629649844	0.470062	-0.488988	
PIK3CA	HCC2157			-0.421896061	0.142	-0.459555	
PIK3CA	ZR7530		-1.212831826	-0.007302976	0.1018	-0.441593	
PIK3CA	**JIMT1**	**-0.902268923**		**0.074417171**	**0.745165**	**-0.337172**	**p.C420R**
PIK3CA	CAL851			0.06175076	0.7936	-0.335181	
PIK3CA	HCC70		-0.029547603	0.556597528	0.6806	-0.322982	
PIK3CA	HCC1806	-0.21067138	-0.180395629	-0.263680183	0.7388	-0.284031	
PIK3CA	**CAL51**	**-1.03325346**	**-0.680618812**	**-0.328897843**	**0.0232**	**-0.202319**	**p.E542K**
PIK3CA	HCC2218		-0.916663045	-1.416569181	0.0448	-0.192815	
PIK3CA	HCC1395	-0.198113287	-0.057281123	0.017833643	0.099596	-0.09432	
PIK3CA	DU4475	-0.151866034		-0.413028823	-0.0049	0.098809	
PIK3CA	**BT483**			**-0.48182782**	**0.3529**	**0.143942**	**p.E542K**
PIK3CA	MDAMB415	-0.065050595	-0.451854236	-0.476275427	0.635502	0.23373	
PIK3CA	HCC1937	-0.180242837	0.001352663	0.230827366	0.9515	0.301673	
PIK3CA	MDA-MB-468	-0.058968772	-0.084448374	-0.712589105	-0.4474	0.305566	
PIK3CA	HCC1419	-0.841580541		-0.352438844	0.1668	0.347683	
PIK3CA	BT549	-0.114036407		0.024376489	-0.0128	0.391756	
PIK3CA	CAMA1	-0.329118351		0.352297907	0.1353	0.418924	
PIK3CA	MDA-MB-231	-0.073360627	-0.146142932	-0.299184538	0.1144	0.424217	
PIK3CA	MDAMB157	-0.225271059	-0.602540222	0.007302976	0.2733	0.526588	
PIK3CA	MDAMB436	-0.166878795	-0.084172255	-0.546295354	-0.6473	0.785837	
PIK3CA	HCC1500		-0.107385257	0.846022069	0.8485	1.01505	
PIK3CA	CAL120		-0.300251542	-0.411261897	0.3055	2.1945	
PIK3CA	HCC1428	-0.179800226	-0.135680755	0.039959305	0.5703	3.109997	

Table 7.4. Relationship between PIK3CA point mutations, essentiality and sensitivity to Alpelisib.

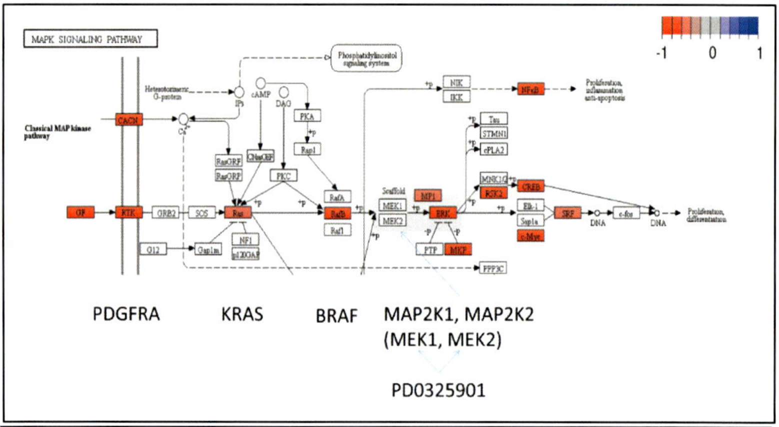

Figure 8.1 Essential genes in DU4475 cell line that map to the MAPK KEGG pathway.

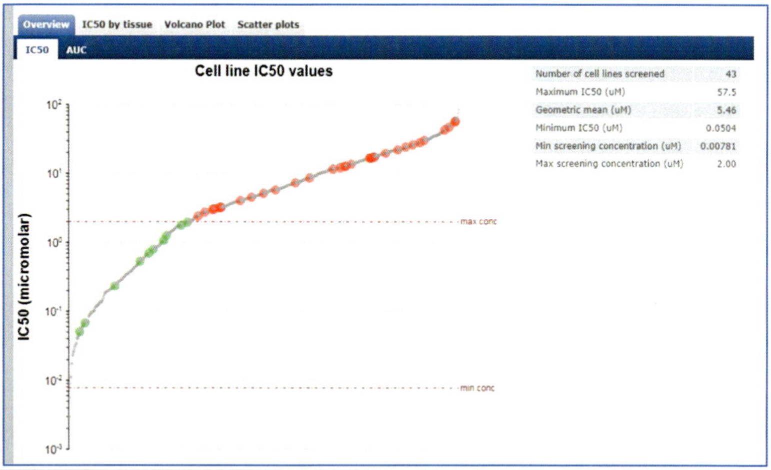

Figure 10.1. Range of sensitivities (IC50s) to Navitoclax for 967 cancer cell lines. The green and red dots show the IC50s for the 43 breast cancer cell lines tested. Note the log scale on the y-axis indicating a nearly 10,000-fold range in sensitivities to this drug for cancer cell lines.

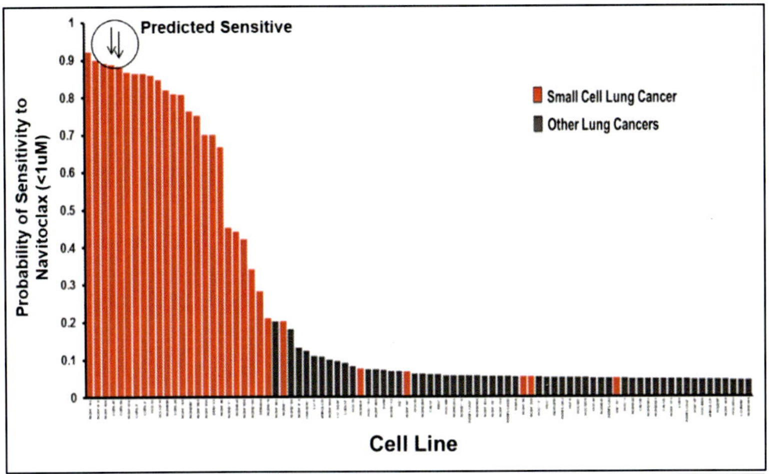

Figure 10.2. Distribution of probabilities of sensitivity to Navitoclax in 86 lung cancer cell lines. Red bars indicate small cell lung cancer lines and black bars indicate non-small cell lung cancer cell lines.

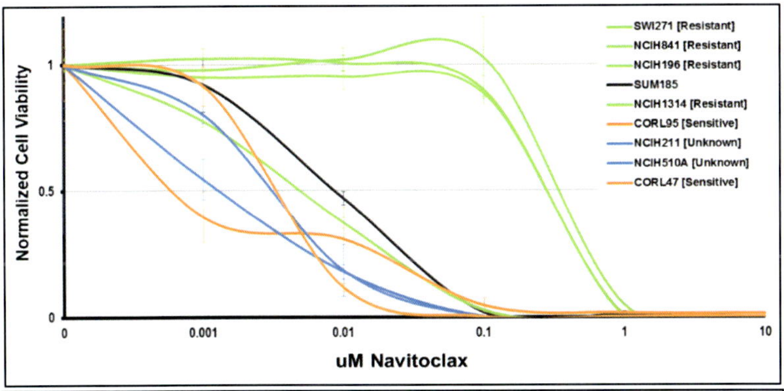

Figure 10.3. IC50 values for nine cancer cell lines treated with Navitoclax. Green lines were derived from small cell lung cancer cell lines that were predicted to be resistant to Navitoclax.

agonist in bone and other tissues. This duality of biological effects results in efficacy at blocking growth and survival of breast cancer cells while providing several desirable side effects, such as maintenance of bone density and low levels of low-density lipoproteins (LDLs) (V.C. Jordan 2006, 2008, 2014, 2021).

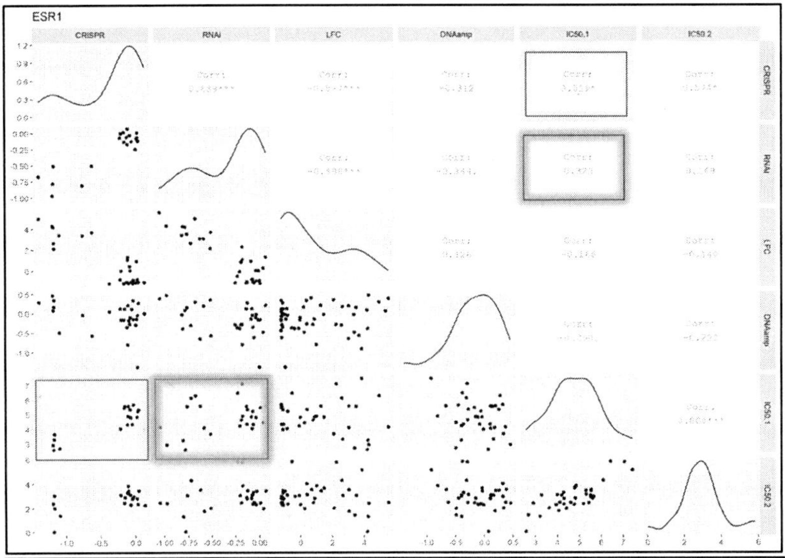

Figure 7.1 Correlation plots for genomic and gene essentiality data for ESR1 in the breast cancer cell line panel. Yellow highlighted box shows the data for the association of CRISPR based essentiality and the IC50 for GDC0810. Blue highlighted boxes show values based on RNAi screen data. *See centrefold for this image in colour.*

For these reasons, TAM is the standard of care for women with ER+ pre-menopausal breast cancer. Beyond Tamoxifen, SERD drugs are commonly used in patients as these drugs degrade the ER and are effective in patients in which ER activity has become estrogen independent. The most commonly used SERD is fulvestrant, but as mentioned earlier, this drug has issues with bioavailability. As a result, new generations of soluble, and thus more bioavailable SERDs are being developed (Manohar and Davidson 2021; Marti and Sanchez-Mendez 2021; Cucciniello et al. 2022).

Variant	Cell.line	CRISPR	RNAi	LFC	DNAamp	Z.score.2
ESR1	**MCF7**	**-1.18036952**	**-0.78112115**	**4.193281236**	**0.072386**	**-2.656779**
ESR1	**CAMA1**	**-1.09084778**		**3.407229827**	**-0.495**	**-2.54482**
ESR1	**EFM19**	**-1.18895946**	**-0.97085516**	**4.292021817**	**0.4591**	**-2.291865**
ESR1	**T47D**		**-0.80228517**	**4.23392322**	**-0.3971**	**-1.967374**
ESR1	**HCC1419**	**-1.17260532**		**2.653920144**	**0.1656**	**-1.884934**
ESR1	**MDAMB415**	**-1.16942107**	**-0.51293873**	**2.102237023**	**0.340575**	**-1.503542**
ESR1	DU4475	0.1362821		-1.099977516	-0.0116	-1.15571
ESR1	AU565	-0.20966055	-0.07515477	-0.832497205	0.1178	-1.08924
ESR1	MDAMB361		-0.58339533	3.039952745	0.1876	-1.028283
ESR1	HCC1500		-1.04369729	5.541605976	0.376	-0.975961
ESR1	MDA-MB-231	-0.1135913	-0.06349525	-1.086680693	-0.3614	-0.785143
ESR1	CAL148			-1.168364491	-0.0825	-0.771152
ESR1	MDAMB157	-0.04612554	-0.12993241	-1.060449152	0.1073	-0.761996
ESR1	CAL851			-0.331303062	-0.3993	-0.670034
ESR1	HCC70		0.041941437	0.258877148	-0.49	-0.647553
ESR1	BT20		-0.18799998	0.79977101	-0.2868	-0.444105
ESR1	HCC1806	-0.19423238	-0.00708035	-0.009374967	-0.176	-0.323748
ESR1	MDA-MB-468	-0.06729578	-0.03570804	0.003115977	-0.1125	-0.26525
ESR1	EFM192A			1.493863136	-0.0379	-0.244697
ESR1	HCC1954	0.024217207	-0.083482	0.893327831	-0.1519	-0.220263
ESR1	HCC1937	-0.10260697	-0.1743028	1.024718231	-0.8104	-0.18249
ESR1	HS578T	0.012036171	-0.24852979	-1.140619501	-0.297437	0.112852
ESR1	CAL51	0.036525054	-0.07110116	-0.799582583	-0.0546	0.192077
ESR1	HDQP1			0.216597344	0.1552	0.220394
ESR1	MDAMB436	0.049717758	-0.12321358	-1.086680693	0.261927	0.322114
ESR1	JIMT1	-0.07650913		0.41659801	-0.276511	0.326364
ESR1	MDAMB453	-0.15852926	0.010744388	-1.196653536	-0.1724	0.458215
ESR1	UACC812		-0.76033225	3.512003568	0.1425	0.548188
ESR1	HCC1395	-0.14797668	-0.13559383	-1.168364491	0.112643	0.563096
ESR1	HCC1143	-0.10144188	0.06837317	1.289793225	0.201385	0.574479
ESR1	BT474		-0.62224052	3.050521987	-0.6621	0.575973
ESR1	HCC2157			-1.196653536	-0.4491	0.636943
ESR1	BT549	-0.02716235		-1.196653536	0.3285	0.695894
ESR1	ZR7530		-0.72129899	2.601489172	-0.3102	1.168363
ESR1	HCC1428	-1.38724254	-0.67275976	4.95450119	0.2831	1.341568
ESR1	CAL120		-0.22626741	-0.52394814	-0.3784	1.544801
ESR1	MDAMB175VII		-0.17796122	2.260178632	-0.2938	2.237782
ESR1	BT483			3.867515617	-0.9192	2.624753

Table 7.1. Relationship between ESR1 expression, essentiality, and sensitivity to GDC0810. *See centrefold for this table in colour.*

For ease of presentation of the results of the analysis in this section, I will start by showing the relationship between one of the newer bio-available SERD drugs, GDC0810 and ESR1 expression and essentiality in the panel of breast cancer cell lines. The rationale for looking at this drug first will become clear momentarily.

Table 7.1 shows the lists of breast cancer cell lines ranked by their Z-scores for GDC0810. Note that the first six rows of this table show the cell lines for which the Z-scores for this drug range from -2.56 to -1.50. Thus, these cell lines are sensitive to this drug. Note also that for all six of these cell lines, ESR1 is highly overexpressed (lfc column) and was highly essential in one or both of the screens. As I indicated above, this is the good news and we will see this same trend in the tables for other targeted drugs that follow.

The next two rows show cell lines that are not sensitive to this drug, which is not surprising because the ESR1 gene is not overexpressed in these cells, nor was the gene found to be essential. But now, look at rows 10 and 11. The MDA-MB-361 and the HCC1500 cell lines overexpress ESR1, and the gene was essential in the screen, and yet these cell lines are not particularly sensitive to GDC0810. Scrolling down the table further reveals five other cell lines that overexpress ESR1, and these cells exhibit varying levels of *resistance* to GDC0810. Examination of the molecular features associated with these less sensitive to resistant cells shows that, of the seven non-sensitive cell lines, five of them have ERBB2 amplifications and three of them have PIK3CA point mutations. One cell line has overexpression of the KRAS gene that was found to be essential in the screen, and these cells also overexpress the BCL2 gene (keep this point in mind for later). Examination of the drug sensitivity data for the HCC1428 cell line shows that these cells seem to be resistant to all targeted drugs tested. This result suggests that the *molecular context* in which ESR1 overexpression occurs has an impact on the effectiveness of this ER-targeted drug, even in the context of high gene essentiality! With respect to ERBB2 amplification in the setting of ER-positivity, it has long been known that patients that are ER+ and ERBB2+ respond less well to ER-targeted drugs than patients without ERBB2 amplifications. Thus, once again the cell line data reflect clinical reality.

Table 7.2 shows the results for a similar analysis for Tamoxifen across the cell line panel. It can be seen from this table that here again, the top three cell lines most sensitive to TAM have ESR1 overexpression associated with gene essentiality. For this drug, however, there are many more ER+

Variant	Cell.line	CRISPR	RNAi	LFC	DNAamp	Z.score.1
ESR1	**T47D**		**-0.802285175**	**4.23392322**	**-0.3971**	**-3.341002**
ESR1	**MCF7**	**-1.18036952**	**-0.781121154**	**4.193281236**	**0.072386**	**-2.217613**
ESR1	**MDAMB361**		**-0.583395334**	**3.039952745**	**0.1876**	**-1.491907**
ESR1	HCC1569		-0.052670392	-1.140619501	-0.6261	-0.976834
ESR1	HCC1428	-1.387242538	-0.672759758	4.95450119	0.2831	-0.921562
ESR1	HCC1954	0.024217207	-0.083482001	0.893327831	-0.1519	-0.892774
ESR1	JIMT1	-0.07650913		0.41659801	-0.276511	-0.86876
ESR1	BT549	-0.02716235		-1.196653536	0.3285	-0.867285
ESR1	HCC1500		-1.043697285	5.541605976	0.376	-0.620545
ESR1	DU4475	0.1362821		-1.099977516	-0.0116	-0.602773
ESR1	EFM19	-1.188959455	-0.970855159	4.292021817	0.4591	-0.579059
ESR1	EFM192A			1.493863136	-0.0379	-0.429355
ESR1	CAL120		-0.226267409	-0.52394814	-0.3784	-0.26218
ESR1	MDAMB415	-1.169421071	-0.512938733	2.102237023	0.340575	-0.07861
ESR1	MDA-MB-468	-0.06729578	-0.035708038	0.003115977	-0.1125	-0.036375
ESR1	HCC1806	-0.194232383	-0.007080352	-0.009374967	-0.176	-0.013609
ESR1	UACC812		-0.760332253	3.512003568	0.1425	0
ESR1	HCC1599			0.402522824	0.3249	0
ESR1	CAL148			-1.168364491	-0.0825	0
ESR1	MDA-MB-231	-0.113591305	-0.063495253	-1.086680693	-0.3614	0.029244
ESR1	CAL51	0.036525054	-0.071101155	-0.799582583	-0.0546	0.053098
ESR1	HCC2157			-1.196653536	-0.4491	0.292693
ESR1	AU565	-0.209660546	-0.075154772	-0.832497205	0.1178	0.413629
ESR1	MDAMB453	-0.158529259	0.010744388	-1.196653536	-0.1724	0.425666
ESR1	MDAMB157	-0.046125536	-0.129932413	-1.060449152	0.1073	0.462591
ESR1	HCC70		0.041941437	0.258877148	-0.49	0.470361
ESR1	HS578T	0.012036171	-0.248529787	-1.140619501	-0.297437	0.525394
ESR1	HDQP1			0.216597344	0.1552	0.644026
ESR1	BT474		-0.62224052	3.050521987	-0.6621	0.695099
ESR1	HCC2218		-0.029199221	-0.972221969	-0.0352	0.716685
ESR1	MDAMB175VII		-0.177961216	2.260178632	-0.2938	0.799203
ESR1	HCC1937	-0.102606973	-0.174302805	1.024718231	-0.8104	0.809213
ESR1	CAMA1	-1.090847779		3.407229827	-0.495	0.818577
ESR1	BT20		-0.187999981	0.79977101	-0.2868	0.820859
ESR1	UACC893			0.695881767	0.387	0.873568
ESR1	HCC1143	-0.101441881	0.06837317	1.289793225	0.201385	0.880904
ESR1	HCC1395	-0.14797668	-0.13559383	-1.168364491	0.112643	0.999166
ESR1	CAL851			-0.331303062	-0.3993	1.042064
ESR1	MDAMB436	0.049717758	-0.123213582	-1.086680693	0.261927	1.156737
ESR1	HCC202	0.035574128	0.003893899	-0.924127681	-1.3869	1.199007
ESR1	HCC1419	-1.17260532		2.653920144	0.1656	1.200606
ESR1	BT483			3.867515617	-0.9192	1.994687
ESR1	ZR7530		-0.721298992	2.601489172	-0.3102	2.20956

Table 7.2. Relationship between ESR1 expression, essentiality and sensitivity to Tamoxifen. *See centrefold for this table in colour.*

cell lines with poor sensitivity to Tamoxifen, particularly as compared to the results with the SERD drug GDC0810. This finding suggests that those cell lines that are sensitive to the SERD drug but not the SERM drug, while requiring functional ER for their growth, do not require estrogen. This is a relatively underappreciated finding and could form the basis for further work on the estrogen-independence in breast cancer.

ERBB2 gene essentiality and targeted drug sensitivity. Now, let's move on to the analysis of the relationship between amplification and essentiality of ERBB2 and sensitivity to the ERBB2-specific tyrosine kinase inhibitor CP724714 (Table 7.3). Once again, as was the case for the ER-targeted drugs, the cells exhibiting the highest sensitivity (lowest Z-scores) to CP724714 can be seen in the top 7 rows of the table, and for six of these cell lines, ERBB2 is amplified, overexpressed and essential in the screens. We will come back to a discussion of that seventh sensitive cell line momentarily.

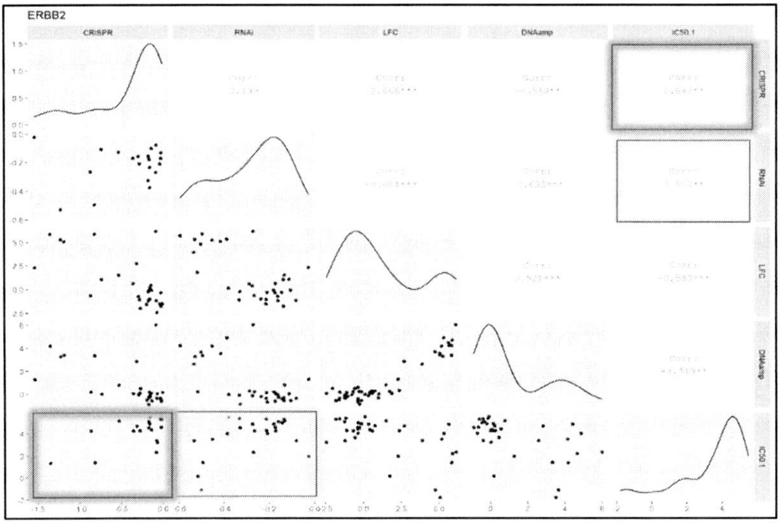

Figure 7.2 Correlation plots for genomic and gene essentiality data for ERBB2 in the breast cancer cell line panel. Blue highlighted box shows the data for the association of CRISPR based essentiality and the IC50 for CP724714. Yellow highlighted boxes show values based on RNAi screen data. *See centrefold for this image in colour.*

As was the case described above, there are four cell lines in which ERBB2 is amplified and overexpressed and yet the cells are not sensitive to the targeted drug. And as was the case for the ER+ cell lines, the ERBB2 amplified but non-sensitive cell lines have other genomic alterations that may help to explain their lack of sensitivity, such as PIK3CA mutations.

But what of the curious case of the MDA-MB-175VII cell line? In this cell line, ERBB2 is not amplified, and only slightly overexpressed. And yet, ERBB2 was found to be essential in this cell line and the cells are highly sensitive to the ERBB2 targeted drug. Does this finding make any sense in terms of the other genomic features of the cell line? Turning to the SLKBase, one can identify some interesting clues that could explain this result. As it happens, MDA-MB175VII is an ER+ cell line, but by transcription profiling, it has been classified as a HER2 subtype cell line,

Variant	Cell.line	CRISPR	RNAi	LFC	DNAamp	CP724714 Z.score.1
ERBB2	HCC2218		-0.412879752	5.085926364	3.5235	-6.512228
ERBB2	BT474		-0.502029224	4.779979821	3.6675	-5.77877
ERBB2	**MDAMB175VII**		**-0.518655663**	**1.761804294**	**0.1792**	**-4.419212**
ERBB2	HCC1419	-1.351421217		5.858527326	4.189	-3.134253
ERBB2	AU565	-0.81489376	-0.495464868	5.854488474	3.3439	-3.095289
ERBB2	MDAMB453	-1.532579796	-0.02423158	2.298230297	1.2681	-2.496664
ERBB2	UACC893			5.899999137	4.6712	-2.238272
ERBB2	DU4475	-0.067051706		-2.433913475	0.019	-1.152206
ERBB2	MDA-MB-468	-0.074025951	-0.079703187	-1.209469731	-0.401	-0.989809
ERBB2	MDAMB361		-0.53421204	3.902117358	2.5961	-0.975548
ERBB2	UACC812		-0.450607423	5.198256237	4.157	-0.858793
ERBB2	CAL851			-0.543207128	0.4595	-0.698149
ERBB2	T47D		-0.286292745	0.560507581	0.2314	-0.325788
ERBB2	HCC1569		-0.384407802	5.340965441	4.8823	-0.292592
ERBB2	HCC1500		-0.207972579	-0.350852711	-0.7226	-0.282167
ERBB2	BT483			2.395847157	0.2715	-0.046626
ERBB2	CAL51	-0.355719982	-0.17093707	0.589073198	0.011	-0.045458
ERBB2	HCC1143	-0.861855521	-0.265565434	-0.66525464	0.170255	-0.044249
ERBB2	MDA-MB-231	-0.275042626	-0.211965409	-1.101676281	0.0894	-0.005125
ERBB2	CAMA1	-0.136003506		0.422877832	0.0638	0.076692
ERBB2	CAL148			1.90295311	0.0148	0.105305
ERBB2	HCC1806	-0.290720436	-0.160191357	-0.761600839	-0.1056	0.119524
ERBB2	HCC1599			-0.355948778	0.5691	0.125323
ERBB2	MCF7	-0.173258166	-0.327824944	-0.257298256	-0.910342	0.267239
ERBB2	HCC1428	-0.019959028	-0.172509257	-0.366880926	-0.6603	0.302553
ERBB2	JIMT1	-0.312425716		2.716116958	2.836604	0.434577
ERBB2	HCC2157			0.770871978	0.2242	0.446333
ERBB2	EFM192A			5.663982249	4.4367	0.592146
ERBB2	BT20		-0.273881933	0.352766186	-0.1969	0.624186
ERBB2	HCC1937	-0.157328692	-0.179569153	-0.127007571	0.1457	0.649099
ERBB2	HCC70		-0.142963938	-0.338695097	-0.4678	0.732642
ERBB2	MDAMB157	-0.168953956	-0.158549776	-1.234905994	-0.3311	0.836555
ERBB2	HS578T	-0.153392581	-0.235331815	-1.032591969	-0.250199	0.884508
ERBB2	EFM19	-0.52682133	-0.130309925	1.501245704	0.779	0.924221
ERBB2	HDQP1			-0.277462708	0.1876	0.962215
ERBB2	MDAMB436	-0.017020248	-0.134415941	-1.807404529	-0.619644	1.092154
ERBB2	HCC1395	-0.028151107	-0.212396361	-1.557616673	-0.415505	1.115574
ERBB2	CAL120		-0.330800845	-1.144537495	-0.1319	1.17848
ERBB2	MDAMB415	-0.152707648	-0.376779018	0.116879292	-0.076872	1.327014

Table 7.3. Relationship between ERBB2 amplification, expression, essentiality and sensitivity to CP724714. *See centrefold for this table in colour.*

which helps to explain the ERBB2 essentiality. Furthermore, this cell line overexpresses ERBB3 and the ERBB3 ligand NRG1 (LFC=4.2 or 16-fold overexpressed). These results suggest that, in this cell line, autocrine activation of ERBB2/ERBB3 plays an important role in the biology of this cell line, both in influencing its transcription profile, and the importance of

ERBB2 signaling in the proliferation of the cells. This finding is potentially very important because it provides our first clue that genomic data may be related to drug sensitivity in a cell line that would not necessarily be predicted based on a single genomic feature. This suggests further that using only a single genomic biomarker for a particular drug can have both false positive and false negative consequences! More on this later.

PIK3CA gene essentiality and targeted drug sensitivity. Finally, let's turn our attention to mutations in PIK3CA and the associations of that genomic feature with essentiality and sensitivity to the targeted drug Alpelisib. As you will see, the story for this gene-drug combination is much the same as described above. Once again, the seven cell lines with the highest sensitivity (lowest Z-scores) to Alpelisib are at the top of the table and all these cell lines have PIK3CA mutations and exhibit high gene essentiality. And, as we saw earlier, scattered throughout the table are seven other cell lines that either have intermediate sensitivity to the Alpelisib or are outright resistant to the drug despite having PIK3CA mutations. Once again, these other cell lines have other genomic features, including PTEN loss, that may play a role in their intrinsic sensitivity to Alelisib.

We have now seen the same story three times. As I mentioned at the outset of this section, the overall correlation coefficients for the relationship between essentiality and drug sensitivity is, at best, around 0.5. And as we have now seen, this is because for each of the genomic features we've looked at, roughly half of the cell lines with the genomic feature are drug sensitive, and the other half exhibit varying levels of sensitivity or resistance.

So, what have we accomplished with this analysis? For one thing, we have shown that for cell lines, like patients, the use of a single genomic feature or biomarker is insufficient to accurately predict targeted drug sensitivity. At best, our predictions might be correct roughly half the time, and that's optimistic. So again, cell lines are people too! Thus, we conclude that essentiality of breast cancer oncogenes in necessary but not sufficient to predict targeted drug sensitivity.

Using gene essentiality data to explore true versus apparent drug resistance. One interesting feature of the results uncovered from this analysis is relevant to the important topic of drug resistance. The presence of intrinsic resistance or acquired resistance to cancer drugs, both traditional chemotherapeutic drugs and targeted drugs, is an important topic in clinical oncology. The results of our analysis allow us to look at this question in a slightly different light. For example, as we have seen, there are cases where cancer cells exhibit a genomic alteration (such as ERBB2 amplification) where there is the expectation that this genomic alteration is associated with drug sensitivity. However, for some of these cell lines, the gene was not found to be essential despite the genomic alteration. In such cases, when it is found that the cells are not sensitive to the targeted drug, the interpretation is usually that the cells are somehow resistant to the drug. However, our analysis argues that the opposite is true, at least in some cases. The lack of essentiality of the gene argues that, rather than the cells being resistant to the drug, there is no reason for the cells to be responsive to the drug in the first place because the genomic alteration in that cell line is not critical to the growth and/or survival of the cancer cells. In this case, the "resistance" is actually an *apparent* resistance and not a *true* resistance and should be recognized as such. By contrast, when we identify cell lines in which the gene, such as ESR1, is highly essential but the cells are still not sensitive to the drug, these are the cases where the basis for the lack of response to the drug needs to be

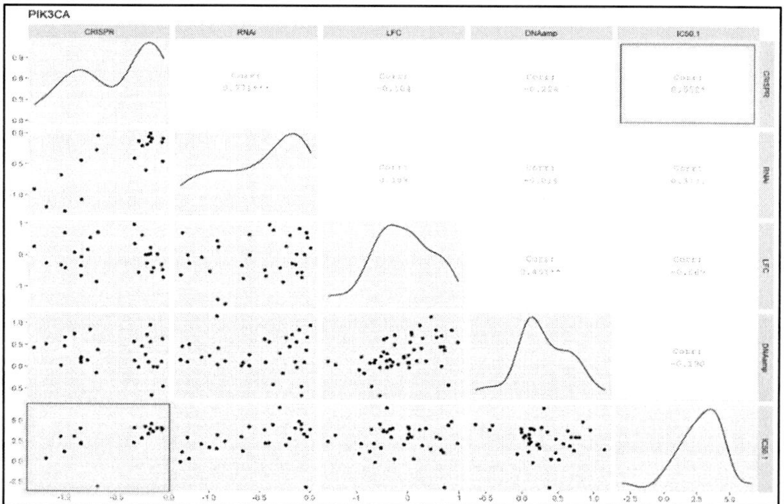

Figure 7.3 Correlation plots for genomic and gene essentiality data for PIK3CA in the breast cancer cell line panel. Yellow highlighted box shows the data for the association of CRISPR based essentiality and the IC50 for Alpelisib. *See centrefold for this image in colour.*

investigated in detail because drug resistance in the context of gene essentiality represents true drug-resistance. There are multiple possible mechanisms for the lack of response to a targeted drug in the context of high gene essentiality. For example, it could be possible that the drug in question is not properly transported into the cell or quickly eliminated. It's possible that the drug-target is not accessible to the drug for other reasons, or the drug does not compete effectively with the ligand for binding to the target. Thus, if one understands as a starting point, the cell lines for which there is a disconnect between essentiality and drug sensitivity, more careful

Variant	Cell.line	CRISPR	RNAi	LFC	DNAamp	Z.score.2	mutation
PIK3CA	MDAMB361		-1.284109778	-0.64251067	0.1533	-2.538572	p.E545K, p.K567R
PIK3CA	MDAMB453	-1.17563853	-1.197997	-0.262086925	0.5131	-2.263952	p.H1047R
PIK3CA	UACC893			0.114218179	0.4061	-2.243956	p.H1047R
PIK3CA	CAL148			-0.958749693	-0.0654	-1.794044	p.D350N, p.H1047R
PIK3CA	BT20		-0.604229288	0.652638094	0.0202	-1.735854	p.P539R, p.H1047R
PIK3CA	EFM19	-0.996488226	-1.267484115	0.69426519	0.4686	-1.680552	p.H1047L
PIK3CA	HCC1954	-0.680242059	-0.038079112	0.713827456	0.3852	-1.472164	p.H1047R
PIK3CA	HCC1599			0.645864866	0.72	-1.471779	
PIK3CA	T47D		-0.922765214	0.447875567	1.1486	-1.378822	p.H1047R
PIK3CA	BT474		-0.994225686	-0.525121331	0.2456	-1.277687	p.K111N
PIK3CA	MDAMB175VII		-0.666812199	-0.745604162	0.0907	-1.172911	
PIK3CA	HCC1569		-0.238750895	0.283052296	0.6627	-1.067204	
PIK3CA	AU565	-0.835473383	-1.075803484	-0.07422691	0.21	-0.987725	
PIK3CA	EFM192A			-0.91803602	0.2292	-0.918925	p.C420R
PIK3CA	MCF7	-0.840496119	-0.440093034	-0.663389399	0.095766	-0.914938	p.E545K
PIK3CA	HS578T	-0.334097503	-0.405952836	0.967113885	0.572631	-0.867087	
PIK3CA	UACC812		-0.841867499	-1.557977159	0.1227	-0.736091	
PIK3CA	HDQP1			-0.089687014	0.2403	-0.531603	
PIK3CA	HCC1143	-0.260664369	-0.20236643	0.629649844	0.470062	-0.488988	
PIK3CA	HCC2157			-0.421896061	0.142	-0.459555	
PIK3CA	ZR7530		-1.212831826	-0.007302976	0.1018	-0.441593	
PIK3CA	JIMT1	-0.902268923		0.074417171	0.745165	-0.337172	p.C420R
PIK3CA	CAL851			0.06175076	0.7936	-0.335181	
PIK3CA	HCC70		-0.029547603	0.556597528	0.6806	-0.322982	
PIK3CA	HCC1806	-0.21067138	-0.180395629	-0.263680183	0.7388	-0.284031	
PIK3CA	CAL51	-1.03325346	-0.680618812	-0.328897843	0.0232	-0.202319	p.E542K
PIK3CA	HCC2218		-0.916663045	-1.416569181	0.0448	-0.192815	
PIK3CA	HCC1395	-0.198113287	-0.057281123	0.017833643	0.099596	-0.09432	
PIK3CA	DU4475	-0.151866034		-0.413028823	-0.0049	0.098809	
PIK3CA	BT483			-0.48182782	0.3529	0.143942	p.E542K
PIK3CA	MDAMB415	-0.065050595	-0.451854236	-0.476275427	0.635502	0.23373	
PIK3CA	HCC1937	-0.180242837	0.001352663	0.230827366	0.9515	0.301673	
PIK3CA	MDA-MB-468	-0.058968772	-0.084448374	-0.712589105	-0.4474	0.305566	
PIK3CA	HCC1419	-0.841580541		-0.352438844	0.1668	0.347683	
PIK3CA	BT549	-0.114036407		0.024376489	-0.0128	0.391756	
PIK3CA	CAMA1	-0.329118351		0.352297907	0.1353	0.418924	
PIK3CA	MDA-MB-231	-0.073360627	-0.146142932	-0.299184538	0.1144	0.424217	
PIK3CA	MDAMB157	-0.225271059	-0.602540222	0.007302976	0.2733	0.526588	
PIK3CA	MDAMB436	-0.166878795	-0.084172255	-0.546295354	-0.6473	0.785837	
PIK3CA	HCC1500		-0.107385257	0.846022069	0.8485	1.01505	
PIK3CA	CAL120		-0.300251542	-0.411261897	0.3055	2.1945	
PIK3CA	HCC1428	-0.179800226	-0.135680755	0.039959305	0.5703	3.109997	

Table 7.4. Relationship between PIK3CA point mutations, essentiality and sensitivity to Alpelisib. *See centrefold for this table in colour.*

and precise experiments can be carried out to understand the basis of targeted drug resistance in individual cell lines. Unfortunately, it is rare for studies on drug resistance to be carried out in the context of an understanding of target gene essentiality and this has resulted in much confusion in the field.

In the next chapter, we will look at one more approach to identifying essential genes that are good druggable targets and will show how sometimes, gene essentiality studies can miss drug-target interactions that are highly potent and specific. If we are to correctly predict all targeted drug sensitivities in patients, it is important that we not miss this important class of essential genes and their cognate drugs to which some cells are highly sensitive.

CHAPTER 8

USING DRUG SENSITIVITY DATA TO IDENTIFY OTHER ESSENTIAL GENES IN BREAST CANCER CELL LINES

We have seen thus far that gene essentiality as determined using either RNAi or CRISPR based drop-out screens provides a window into the potential for genes to be good druggable targets. We have also seen that even for essential genes, drug sensitivity doesn't always follow directly from essentiality. The question now is whether the opposite might also be true. That is, are there genes that do not score as essential in either type of drop-out assay that are nonetheless good drug targets associated with high drug sensitivity in certain specific contexts?

To address this question, all one has to do as a starting point is to consult the Genomics of Drug Sensitivity in Cancer database and examine any number of cell lines and look at the rank ordered list of the drugs to which each cell line is most sensitive. As I have examined these results, I have noted that it is not unusual to see high drug sensitivities associated with genes that weren't found to be essential in drop-out screens. However, there is an important caveat to this type of cursory analysis.

Recently, a paper was published by Lin and co-workers (Lin et al. 2019) at Cold Spring Harbor laboratory. These investigators were interested in a particular drug to which several cell lines were highly sensitive and for which the targets of the drugs were known, or at least, presumed to be known. When these investigators performed targeted knock-out experiments of the putative target genes using different CRISPR base sgRNA vectors, they consistently found that the presumed target gene of the drug was not essential in any of the drug-sensitive cell lines. One possible conclusion of this result is that the presumed targets of the drugs are not the correct targets at all. To investigate this possibility further, they performed mutagenesis experiments in the sensitive cell lines and identified variants that had acquired resistance to a targeted drug. Then, they identified the mutations that occurred commonly in the resistant variants that were associated with the acquired resistance. Using this approach, the team identified the correct target of the drug by identifying the gene that was commonly mutated in the newly drug resistant cell line variants. As part of this report, the authors found that this type of target misidentification is not uncommon and is associated with poor results in clinical trials of targeted drugs.

This important finding indicates that one must proceed with caution when attempting to make the connection between drug sensitivity and a particular target, especially when the presence or genomic state of the target is used as a predictive biomarker for drug sensitivity. If the target-biomarker is not correct, then patient selection for clinical trials cannot be done correctly, and as a result, these trials will yield a negative result. Knowing the true and correct target for a drug is, therefore, necessary for proper design and execution of any clinical trial involving a targeted drug.

By contrast to this story, there are examples in the GDSC database for which drug sensitivity in the absence of gene essentiality still points to correct drug-target interactions. One excellent example of this can be observed when looking at the genomic data, gene essentiality data, and drug sensitivity data for the DU4475 breast cancer cell line.

The DU4475 breast cancer cell line was derived from a metastatic skin nodule of a 62-year-old Caucasian patient previously diagnosed with breast cancer. Genomic analysis of this cell line along with gene essentiality data show that this skin-derived cell line has the classic V600E point mutation in the BRAF oncogene. Furthermore, BRAF was found to be highly essential (CERES score -1.7) in the CRISPR based drop out screen in this cell line. By now, it is well known that the V600E point mutation in the BRAF oncogene occurs in roughly 50% of melanomas and when this mutation is present, cells and patients are highly sensitive to and responsive to the BRAF-targeted drug Vemurafenib and other similar BRAF targeted drugs. Thus, it is not surprising that DU4475 cells are also highly sensitive to not only Vemurafenib (Z-score -3.29) but also to two different BRAF targeted drugs. Thus, for these cells, BRAF is a functional driving oncogene to which there is a strong connection between the genomic alteration, gene essentiality, and drug sensitivity.

Now, when one examines the drug sensitivity data for DU4475 cell line in the GDSC database, one is immediately struck by the sensitivity of these cells to another drug, PD0325901 (Z-score -3.12!). PD0325901 is a MAP Kinase inhibitor that has as its targets the MEK1 and MEK2 proteins that are part of the MAP Kinase signal transduction pathway. The genes that code for MEK1 and MEK2 are MAP2K1 and MAP2K2 respectively. Inspection of the gene essentiality data for these genes shows clearly that neither one of them came close to scoring as hits in the CRISPR screen. So then, how does one explain the disconnect between drug sensitivity and gene essentiality in this case? And do the drug sensitivity data indicate a true on-target effect of the drug? Or could it be that for this drug, the target is also incorrect? This would appear to be unlikely as this drug, and others like it, have been extensively validated for target specificity.

The answer to this question can be observed by looking at the KEGG pathway shown in Figure 8.1. The figure shows the part of the KEGG Map kinase pathway that centers around the BRAF oncogene. The boxes shown in red indicate the genes in this pathway that scored as hits in the CRISPR screen for DU4475. (The KEGG pathway engine on the SLKBase allows users to map all screen hit genes onto any KEGG pathway, and this was used to generate the figure below.) This figure shows that most of the genes in this pathway are essential in this cell line, with several genes both upstream and downstream of the BRAF oncogene scoring as hits in the screens. By contrast, MEK1 and MEK2, which are immediately downstream of BRAF, were not screen hits. The genomic data also show that both of these genes are expressed at normal levels in these cells, and this is key. One can also see from the pathway that the function of BRAF is to phosphorylate MEK1 and MEK2. This phosphorylation event is necessary to activate the MEK kinases and propagate the signal downstream. Finally, what is evident from this figure is that MEK1 and MEK2 have redundant functions and that the drug PD0325901 inhibits the activity of *both kinases*. By contrast, as we have seen, the CRISPR or RNAi based gene essentiality screens can only knock-out or knock-down *one gene at a time* in any given cell. Thus, it is the redundancy of the MAP2K1 and MAP2K2 genes that results in neither gene scoring as hits in the screen because when one gene is knocked down or knocked out, the other isoform still performs the signal transduction function. But when a drug is used that can inactivate *both* kinases, the exquisite sensitivity of the cells to the drug is revealed. Thus, the high sensitivity of this particular drug is a correct on-target effect.

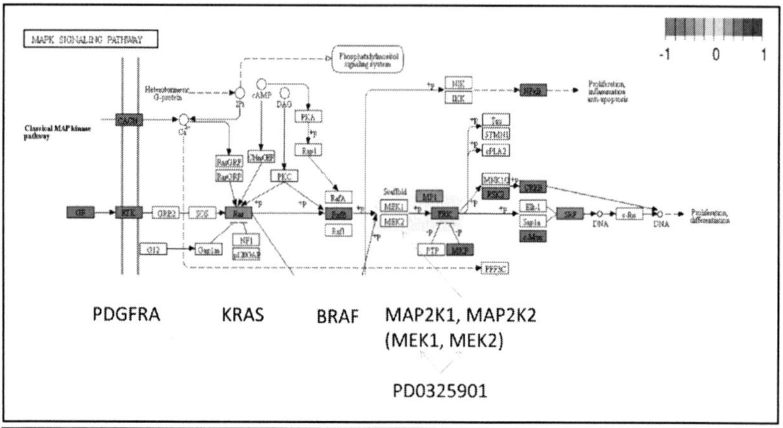

Figure 8.1 Essential genes in DU4475 cell line that map to the MAPK KEGG pathway. *See centrefold for this image in colour.*

This example is illustrative of the factors that one can use to determine if the drug sensitivity data present in the GDSC database represents true on-target drug sensitivities. We have used these factors to develop an algorithm that allows us to identify the drug sensitivities in any cell line that are most likely to be correct on-target drug sensitivities even when there is a disconnect between drug sensitivity and gene essentiality. As will be shown in the next chapter, we have developed drug sensitivity signatures for the 40 breast cancer cell lines described in the SLKBase. Part of those signatures show the drugs to which a given cell line is sensitive based on correct on-target sensitivity despite negative gene essentiality data. To identify the drug sensitivity data that are most likely to represent correct on-target interactions when there is a disconnect with gene essentiality data, we put the following restrictions on the drug sensitivity data present in the GDSC database.

First, we require that a given drug to which a cell line is highly sensitive has more than one target with redundant function, both of which are expressed in the cell line of interest. Such cases make these drugs similar to the MEK1/MEK2 targeted drug PD0325901 described above. The second restriction we place on the data is that the cells exhibit similar sensitivity to more than one drug that has the same target. Small molecule inhibitors are developed independently of each other and so when two structurally different small molecule drugs that were developed against the same target show similar high sensitivities, it is likely that these sensitivities also represent true on target effects regardless of gene essentiality. As will be seen in the next chapter, incorporating this type of analysis into the genomic, gene essentiality and drug sensitivity data enriches the drug sensitivity signatures for the cell lines in our database.

As a result of the work presented thus far, we now have everything we need to build targeted drug sensitivity signatures for any cancer cell line for which functional genomics and drug sensitivity data are available. In the next chapter, I will illustrate how these data are used to build these signatures and the kinds of predictions they make for representative cell lines.

CHAPTER 9

USING FUNCTIONAL GENOMICS TO DEFINE DRUG SENSITIVITY SIGNATURES FOR BREAST CANCER CELL LINES: THE THREE TIERS OF TARGETED DRUG SENSITIVITY

As the title of this book indicates, a primary goal of our work is to develop precision targeted drug strategies that can be used to attack any breast cancer cell line in a manner that is specific to that line. Such an approach can be thought of as reverse engineering a cancer cell line because it is based on a deep understanding of the genes and pathways that drive the oncogenic potential of the cells and linking that knowledge to sensitivity to a panel of targeted drugs that can be used either singly, or in combinations.

To accomplish this goal, we have developed a functional genomics strategy that connects oncogene activation (particularly druggable oncogenes), gene essentiality, and targeted drug sensitivity to identify on a cell line by cell line basis, the drugs that are most likely to reverse the oncogenic potential of the cell line. Using this strategy, we determine for every cell line three tiers of drug sensitivity each of which have different but related underlying rationales.

Tier 1 drug sensitivities are based on the presence, in any given cell line, of functional (essential) druggable oncogenes present in the cell line and determining which oncogene targeted drugs the cells are most sensitive to. Tier 2 drug sensitivities are based on the presence of essential and druggable genes (not oncogenes) that have targeted drugs to which the cells exhibit high sensitivity. Thus, in Tier 2, we identify non-oncogenes where there is a strong connection between gene essentiality and targeted drug sensitivity. Tier 3 signatures show the drugs to which the cells are highly sensitive when there is a **disconnect** between sensitivity and essentiality, and for these cases, we use the restrictions described in the previous chapter to ensure that drug sensitivity is associated with a true on-target effect. Using this approach, we have developed Tier 1, Tier 2, and Tier 3 drug sensitivity signatures for the 40 breast cancer cell lines in our database. As may be obvious by now, using the database and methods we've developed, one need only to expand the scope of the database to include all genomic, functional genomic, and drug sensitivity data for all types of cancer cell lines to allow for the generation of specific reverse engineering strategies for hundreds of cancer cell lines. This is achievable because all the functional genomic data for hundreds of cancer cell lines are publicly available.

Drug sensitivity signatures for representative breast cancer cell lines. To illustrate how our method provides individualized drug sensitivity signatures for breast cancer cell lines, I will describe a few representative examples for cell lines currently on the SLKBase. Note that the drug sensitivity signatures for all 40 breast cancer cell lines are currently present on the SLKBase and can be viewed here https://sumlineknowledge base.com/?page_id=3380 .

The AU565 Breast Cancer Cell Line. The AU565 cell line was derived from the same patient that gave rise to the more famous SKBR3 cell line. As such, both lines are characterized by an ERBB2 (HER2) gene amplification and TP53 mutation. The cell line was derived from a pleural effusion metastasis of a patient diagnosed with breast adenocarcinoma.

The Tier 1, 2 and 3 drug sensitivities for this cell line are shown below. First, note that for this cell line, ERBB2 is a functional driving oncogene because it is amplified, overexpressed, and is associated with high sensitivity to the ERBB2 specific tyrosine kinase inhibitor CP724714 (This drug was only tested for the GDSC1 data set). That this finding represents true on-target drug sensitivity for this oncogene is clear because these cells show high sensitivity to five other ERBB2 targeted drugs. In this regard, it is particularly noteworthy that this cell line exhibits good sensitivity to Lapatinib. Recall from the previous discussion that Lapatinib is a dual specificity inhibitor that targets both ERBB2 and EGFR and, as can be seen in the Tier 3 signature, EGFR is also overexpressed in this cell line. Thus, the sensitivity to Lapatinib makes biological sense in this context. Note that not all ERBB2 amplified breast cancer cell lines exhibit sensitivity to Lapatinib. Thus, the functional genomics signature for AU565 provides a window into the factors that predict sensitivity to this FDA approved drug.

Tier1: AU565								
Drug name	**Gene symbol_HGNC**	**z_score_GDSC1**	**z_score_GDSC2**	**DNA_amp**	**expression**	**mutation**	**COSMIC_hit**	
Lapatinib	ERBB2	0	-2.145526	3.3439	5.854488474	NULL	0	
Afatinib	ERBB2	-2.364684	-2.035281	3.3439	5.854488474	NULL	0	
Sapitinib	ERBB2	0	-1.682239	3.3439	5.854488474	NULL	0	
CP724714	ERBB2	-3.095289	0	3.3439	5.854488474	NULL	0	
CI-1033	ERBB2	-3.460803	0	3.3439	5.854488474	NULL	0	
PF-00299804	ERBB2	-3.999264	0	3.3439	5.854488474	NULL	0	
Tier2: AU565								
Drug name	**Gene symbol_HGNC**	**z_score_GDSC1**	**z_score_GDSC2**	**DNA_amp**	**expression**	**mutation**	**CERES-CRISPR**	**CERES-RNAi**
Rapamycin	MTOR	0	-2.082992	-0.1194	0.095132459	NULL	-1.301219832	-0.917731707
AT13148	AKT1	0	-1.930824	0.3319	0.652507231	NULL	-0.198463775	-0.537905343
Uprosertib	AKT1	0	-1.701098	0.3319	0.652507231	NULL	-0.198463775	-0.537905343
Sapitinib	ERBB3	0	-1.682239	0.0815	0.895966234	p.E952Q	-1.047871935	-0.870693342
AKT inhibitor VIII	AKT1	-2.250084	0	0.3319	0.652507231	NULL	-0.198463775	-0.537905343
Tier3: AU565								
Drug Name	**Gene SymbolHGNC**	**z_score_GDSC1**	**z_score_GDSC2**	**DNA_amp**	**expression**	**mutation**	**CERES-CRISPR**	**CERES RNAi**
MN-64	TNKS	0	-2.620924	-0.7706	-0.033519801	NULL	-0.160955435	-0.214222869
MN-64	TNKS2	0	-2.620924	-0.7996	-0.389591804	NULL	-0.175249976	-0.202173515
Lapatinib	EGFR	0	-2.145526	0.8119	1.361440138	p.R309G	0.07931304	-0.08454952
Afatinib	EGFR	-2.364684	-2.035281	0.8119	1.361440138	p.R309G	0.07931304	-0.08454952
GSK1904529A	IGF1R	-2.297279	-1.670365	-0.2683	-0.571973914	NULL	0.103843149	-0.001585228
GSK1904529A	INSR	-2.297279	-1.670365	-0.6802	-0.470097197	p.V615F	-0.044696116	0.013883225
LGK974	PORCN	-2.52058	-0.541474	0.5131	0.02713613	NULL	0.240630376	0.15117195
Wnt-C59	PORCN	-2.355176	-0.130387	0.5131	0.02713613	NULL	0.240630376	0.15117195
AKT inhibitor VIII	AKT1	-2.250084	0	0.3319	0.652507231	NULL	-0.198463775	-0.537905343
AKT inhibitor VIII	AKT2	-2.250084	0	-0.244	-0.324320939	NULL	-0.341700871	-0.42961282
AKT inhibitor VIII	AKT3	-2.250084	0	0.0732	-1.494182941	NULL	0.076937914	0.108775863
CI-1033	EGFR	-3.460803	0	0.8119	1.361440138	p.R309G	0.07931304	-0.08454952
PF-00299804	EGFR	-3.999264	0	0.8119	1.361440138	p.R309G	0.07931304	-0.08454952
AST-1306	EGFR	-3.801252	0	0.8119	1.361440138	p.R309G	0.07931304	-0.08454952
CI-1033	ERBB4	-3.460803	0	-0.3226	-0.129676307	NULL	-0.081479023	-0.091483524
PF-00299804	ERBB4	-3.999264	0	-0.3226	-0.129676307	NULL	-0.081479023	-0.091483524
AST-1306	ERBB4	-3.801252	0	-0.3226	-0.129676307	NULL	-0.081479023	-0.091483524

Table 9.1 Tier 1, 2 and 3 drug sensitivity signatures for the ERBB2 amplified and TP53 mutant AU565 cell line.

As discussed earlier in this book, it is well known that the ERBB2 oncogene signals primarily through the PI3'kinase pathway. Given that, it is not surprising that in Tier 2, we see that the cells are sensitive to several drugs that target other components of this pathway, including AKT1, MTOR and ERBB3, and all three of these genes scored as hits in both functional screens. Thus, this is Tier 2 drug sensitivity where there is a connection between gene essentiality and targeted drug sensitivity for non-oncogenes that, in this case, are in the same pathway as the main driving oncogene.

Finally, in Tier 3, we see that AU565 cells also exhibit high sensitivity to other drugs that target genes that are primarily related to signaling via other ERBB family members or parts of the PI3'Kinase pathway. In each case the listed drugs either target two or more proteins that are expressed in the cells (as noted in the column labeled 'expression') or there are multiple drugs to the same target to which the cells are sensitive.

As is often the case with Tier 3 drugs, there are caveats that need to be considered for some of the drug sensitivities listed. For example, one can see that the AU565 cells are highly sensitive to a drug called MN-64 that targets the tankerase genes TNKS and TNKS2. Both genes are expressed at near normal levels in these cells. This suggests that this sensitivity represents true on-target activity of MN-64. In another example, a very interesting gene called PORCN is shown to be a good target as the cells are sensitive to two different drugs to the same target. This is particularly intriguing because PORCN is a gene that is an important driver of the WNT signaling pathway that has been long known to be important in cancer. The caveat here though is that both drugs were tested in the development of both the GDSC1 and GDSC2 data sets and the Z-scores (and IC50s) for these drugs are quite different in the two data sets. Some consider the GDSC2 data set to be the more reliable and this casts some doubt on the low Z-score reported in the GDSC1 data set. Thus, one should proceed with caution when interpreting the data for these two targeted drugs. We maintain them in the Tier 3 signature because, at least for the GDSC1 data, the two drugs meet the criteria that we set for Tier 3 drugs. At this time, there is no way to tell which Z-score is correct for these two drugs. Independent verification needs to be carried out to act as a tiebreaker for this drug-cell line interaction. As we will see, there are other examples like this where there is significant disagreement between drug sensitivities displayed in GDSC1 versus GDSC2.

The HCC1419 Breast Cancer Cell Line. The HCC1419 breast cancer cell line was derived from the primary ductal carcinoma a 42-year-old female of European-American and Native American decent. The cell line is both ER-positive and ERBB2 positive. ERBB2 (HER2) is amplified, overexpressed and was a strong hit in the functional screen and the ESR1 gene is highly overexpressed and essential in these cells. Thus, this cell line is similar to AU565 with regard to the ERBB2 amplification but is otherwise different in that it is an ER-positive luminal breast cancer cell line. Thus, the drug sensitivity signature for this line bears both similarities and differences from that of the AU565 cell line.

The Tier 1 drug sensitivity signature shows that, as expected for an ERBB2 amplified cell line in which the gene is highly overexpressed, the cells are highly sensitive to CP724714 as well as two other ERBB2 targeted drugs. Thus, once again, ERBB2 is a functional-druggable oncogene in this cell line. One also sees that the ESR1 gene (ERα) is highly overexpressed in these cells, and we discussed earlier how for this gene, overexpression is always associated with essentiality. In this case, one can see that the cells are quite sensitive to the SERD drug GDC0810, again as expected for a highly ERα positive cell line. Interestingly, RET is also a functional druggable oncogene in this cell line. The RET gene is highly overexpressed in these cells, and they are quite sensitive to the RET targeted drug Motesanib. This finding was unexpected and serves to illustrate how an unbiased analysis of functional genomics data can lead to unexpected but potentially important findings regarding drug sensitivities.

HCC1419.T1									
Drug name	Gene symbol_HGNC	z_score_GDSC1	z_score_GDSC2	DNA_amp	Expression	mutation	COSMIC_hit		
GDC0810	ESR1	0	-1.884934	0.1656	2.653920144	NULL	0		
Motesanib	RET	-2.204144	0	-0.0964	2.958744798	NULL	0		
PF-00299804	ERBB2	-2.911448	0	4.189	5.858527326	NULL	0		
CI-1033	ERBB2	-2.464143	0	4.189	5.858527326	NULL	0		
CP724714	ERBB2	-3.134253	0	4.189	5.858527326	NULL	0		
HCC1419.T2									
Drug name	Gene symbol_HGNC	z_score_GDSC1	z_score_GDSC2	DNA_amp	Expression	mutation	COSMIC_hit	CERES-CRISPR	CERES-RNAI
GDC0810	ESR1	0	-1.884934	0.1656	2.653920144	NULL	0	-1.17260532	NULL
ML323	WDR48	0	-1.574182	0.1236	0.444018966	NULL	0	-0.926235754	NULL
HCC1419.T3									
Drug name	Gene SymbolHGNC	z_score_GDSC1	z_score_GDSC2	DNA_amp	Expression	mutation	COSMIC_hit	achilles_score	demeter
CI-1033	EGFR	-2.464143	0	0.3076	-3.579209641	NULL	0	0.154432175	NULL
PF-00299804	EGFR	-2.911448	0	0.3076	-3.579209641	NULL	0	0.154432175	NULL
AST-1306	EGFR	-2.930609	0	0.3076	-3.579209641	NULL	0	0.154432175	NULL
CI-1033	ERBB4	-2.464143	0	-0.2003	1.996747056	NULL	0	-0.165461749	NULL
PF-00299804	ERBB4	-2.911448	0	-0.2003	1.996747056	NULL	0	-0.165461749	NULL
AST-1306	ERBB4	-2.930609	0	-0.2003	1.996747056	NULL	0	-0.165461749	NULL
Motesanib	KDR	-2.204144	0	0.1337	-0.013939191	NULL	0	0.019017614	NULL
Motesanib	KIT	-2.204144	0	0.1337	0.059177678	NULL	0	-0.266232889	NULL
Motesanib	PDGFRA	-2.204144	0	0.1337	-0.041027268	NULL	0	-0.199950124	NULL
Motesanib	PDGFRB	-2.204144	0	-0.3102	-0.187278568	NULL	0	0.029946875	NULL
Motesanib	RET	-2.204144	0	-0.0964	2.958744798	NULL	0	0.062279488	NULL

Table 9.2 Tier 1, 2 and 3 drug sensitivity signatures for the ERBB2 amplified and ER+ cell line HCC1419.

The Tier 2 drug sensitivity signature shows that, in addition to GDC0810 that targets ERα, the cells are moderately sensitive to a drug called ML323 that targets a gene called WDR48. WDR48 interacts with ubiquitin specific peptidase (USP1) and that interaction activates the deubiquitinating activity of USP1. There is evidence to suggest that the deubiquitinating activity of the WDR48/USP1 complex maintains cancer stem cells in an undifferentiated state. Thus, inhibiting that activity may be effective to treat cancer stem cells (Goncalves, Cordeiro, and Rivero 2017). This drug sensitivity appears in this signature because WDR48 was a hit in the CRISPR screen. This then is another unexpected finding that results from our functional genomic analysis of drug sensitivity.

The Tier 3 signature once again identifies other less specific drugs that target members of the ERBB family to which the cells are quite sensitive. But, noteworthy in its absence here is Lapatinib, and one can see from the Tier 3 table that EGFR is not expressed in these cells. The lack of EGFR expression is consistent with the ERα positivity of this cell line. Note that the drug Motesanib also appears in the Tier 3 signature because this drug is a multi-kinase inhibitor that targets other signaling molecules beyond RET, but only RET is overexpressed in these cells.

These results are a good starting point to highlight the importance of developing individual reverse engineering strategies for every cell line based on their particular functional genomic attributes rather than trying to group cell lines or patients based on an individual genomic feature such as ERBB2 amplification or ESR1 overexpression. It is particularly noteworthy that even though these cells are ERBB2 amplified, Lapatinib did not appear in any of the drug sensitivity tiers for this cell line. Indeed, by consulting the Functional Druggable Signature tool on the SLKBase, one can see that these cells are actually quite resistant to Lapatinib.

Other interesting features of drug signatures for cell lines. One thing comes into clearer focus as one starts to examine specific drug sensitivity signatures for individual breast cancer cell lines. That is, as we have been saying all along, breast cancer cell lines are unique representations of the disease from which the cell line was derived, and thus, drug sensitivity signatures are as unique as the cell lines themselves. Thus, there is no one -size-fits-all for predicting drug sensitivity based on simple characteristics of the cancer cells. To illustrate this point further, I will point out some interesting features of the drug signatures of other breast cancer cell lines, and I will provide links to those signatures so that the details can be viewed on the SLKBase.

Let's begin with the CAL51 cell line (https://sumlineknowledgebase.com/?page_id=3399). This cell line is classified as a Basal B triple negative breast cancer. Despite its triple negativity, this line has a PIK3CA point mutation as well as a mutation in the PTEN tumor suppressor gene. Thus, in this line, there are two distinct genomic alterations that result in constitutive activation of the PI3'Kinase pathway. Given the presence of the PTEN mutation coincident with the PIK3CA mutation, it might not be surprising to find that the cells are not particularly sensitive to PIK3CA inhibitors as none of these drugs appear in the Tier1 signature. Indeed, by consulting the Functional Druggable Signature tool on the SLKBase, one can see that the Z-score for Alpelisib is -0.202 meaning that the cells are no more sensitive to this drug than the average of all cell lines. The cells are more responsive to a less isoform specific PI3'K targeted drug, Dactolisib, but even here the Z-score is only -1.10 indicating moderate sensitivity. Thus, the presence of the PTEN mutation in this cell line appears to blunt the effectiveness of PIK3CA targeted drugs. This is not surprising because PTEN is a strong negative regulator of PI3'K activity the function of which is lost in these cells. Thus, when PTEN is inactive, PI3'kinase activity can persist even when the kinase activity of PIK3CA is attenuated with a targeted drug.

While this is discouraging, one can also see in the Tier 2 signature that these cells have good sensitivity to two cell-cycle targeted drugs, PLK1 and ATR. Both genes were screen hits and the Z-scores for both drugs are less than the cut-point of -1.5. I illustrate this here because we have found that triple negative breast cancer cell lines often exhibit sensitivity to drugs that target PLK1 or ATR. Finally, CAL51 cells show high sensitivity to two different PARP1/2 targeted drugs. This is significant because this cell line does not have a BRCA1/2 mutation, and thus one would not automatically consider PARP inhibitors as being effective for this cell line, but the empirical data suggest otherwise.

Thus, even though CAL51 is an aggressive Basal B cell line, there are several targeted drugs to which the cells are highly sensitive, none of which would be immediately obvious just by knowing the cells are PIK3CA and PTEN mutant or are Basal B type breast cancer cells.

Next let's consider the BT20 cell line (https://sumlineknowledgebase.com/?page_id=3481). This cell line has traditionally been used to study the role of EGFR signaling in breast cancer cells because the cells exhibit amplification and overexpression of the EGFR gene. These cells also have a PIK3CA mutation, so there are two potential functional druggable oncogenes in this cell line. I demonstrated in an earlier chapter that EGFR gene amplification/overexpression is not a predictor of essentiality or sensitivity to any of the EGFR-targeted *small molecule* drugs. However, examination of the Tier 1 drug signature for BT20 cells reveals a surprise. Whereas these cells are not sensitive to any of the small molecule inhibitors of EGFR signaling, these cells are highly sensitive to the drug Cetuximab, which is an antibody-based drug that targets EGFR! Interestingly, essentially the same result was obtained using the only other breast cancer cell line with an EGFR gene amplification, MDA-468. For these cells as well, there is no significant sensitivity to small molecule EGFR targeted drugs, but the Tier 1 signature for MDA-468 also indicates good sensitivity to Cetuximab.

This is fascinating in light of the fact that the first clinically useful ERBB2 (HER2) targeted drug was, and is, Trastuzumab, which is also an antibody type of drug. And indeed, the small molecule ERBB2 inhibitors that were developed later were found to be less effective in patients than the antibody-type drug(s). These results suggest that for growth factor receptors such as EGFR and ERBB2, using antibodies to block their activity is superior to using kinase inhibitors to block activity, even in an *in vitro* setting. These are findings that would not have been predicted but tell us something about the best ways to inhibit signaling from overexpressed cell surface receptors.

Finally, as indicated above, BT20 cells have a PIK3CA mutation and the cells are sensitive to Alpelisib, which appears in the Tier 1 drug signature. Thus, both functional-druggable oncogenes are targetable in this cell line, and the signatures tell us precisely which drugs against these targets are going to be most effective.

The CAL120 cell line (https://sumlineknowledgebase.com/?page_id=3487) is another Basal B triple negative breast cancer cell line, and like most such lines, the oncogene signature doesn't tell us anything about drug sensitivity. However, examination of the Tier 2 signature for this cell line shows that BCL2L1 is a good target in these cells as the gene was a strong hit in both screens, and the cells are highly sensitive to the BCL2L1 targeted drug, WEHI-539. Once again, other than this type of empirical determination, there would have been no other way to predict the sensitivity of these cells to a BCL2L1 targeted drug. Given that this is a Basal B triple negative cell line that most people assume are devoid of drug targets, knowing the essentialness of BCL2L1 and the sensitivity to WEHI-539 provides a novel insight into a reverse engineering strategy for this cell line.

I will close this section with a discussion of two ER+ breast cancer cell lines. The EFM19 cell line overexpresses the ESR1 gene, which as we have mentioned is highly essential in these cells. These cells also have a PIK3CA mutation. Given the ERα positivity and essentialness of ESR1, it is not surprising that the cells are sensitive to the SERD drug GDC0810. Thus, these sensitivities present opportunities for interesting drug combinations, and this will be discussed on more detail in the next chapter. Examination of the Tier 2 and Tier 3 drug sensitivity signatures of this cell line shows that, not surprisingly for a line with a PIK3CA mutation, the cells are also sensitive to drugs that target other members of the PI3'Kinase family, and the Tier 3 signature shows that these cells are sensitive to two different drugs that target genes in the apoptotic pathway: BIRC3, XIAP, and NAIP. Thus, there are myriad possible way to attack and reverse engineer this cell line based on these functional genomics data

The CAMA1 cell line is an example of an ER-positive cell line that also has an amplification of the 8p11 genomic region, which is fairly common in aggressive ER-positive breast cancer. That said, this genomic region does not present any druggable targets associated with drug sensitivity (including FGFR1 as we discussed previously). However, we find from examining the Tier 1 signature that the cells are highly sensitive to the SERD drug GDC0810, but also the androgen receptor targeted drug, Bicalutamide, as the androgen receptor is highly overexpressed in these cells. The Tier 3 signature also points to active signaling through the PI3'Kinase pathway even in the absence of PIK3CA or PTEN mutations, as the cells are very sensitive to several drugs that target different members of this pathway.

Once again, the upshot of all this is that cell lines are people too, and it is not possible to predict strategies to reverse engineer individual cell lines in a manner that is simple and straight forward. The question then is this, is such individuality a feature or a bug? Most in our field would throw their hands up at seeing this and conclude that there is no future for targeted therapy because it seems to be impossible to predict drug sensitivity in an individual patient. However, as I will attempt to show in coming chapters, the individuality in drug sensitivity signatures is actually the key to the ultimate development of truly personalized and precise drug strategies for breast cancer, particularly for patients with metastatic disease.

CHAPTER 10

ARTIFICIAL INTELLIGENCE AND MACHINE LEARNING METHODS TO PREDICT TARGETED DRUG SENSITIVITY IN PATIENTS

We have now seen how functional genomic data can be used to identify the most essential genes in any cancer-derived cell line, determine which of them are activated oncogenes, which of them are druggable and associated with drug sensitivity, and how to identify other targeted drugs based on their on-target sensitivity. As we have seen, all of this has allowed us to develop Tier 1, Tier 2, and Tier 3 drug sensitivity signatures for over 40 breast cancer cell lines. We will soon be applying this strategy to develop similar drug sensitivity signatures for hundreds of other cancer cell lines of many different types. In the next chapter, we will show how it is possible to leverage drug sensitivity data to identify drug combinations that may act in synergy to induce cancer cell-specific lethality.

This would be all well and good if the goal was to cure cancer cell lines. But obviously that is not the goal. Thus, we must now address the question of how one can use these functional data sets in a way that yields practical benefit to patients in real life. It should be obvious by now that what we have generated so far, and what we are continuing to build, is a large functional genomics database. Queries of that relational database can be quickly and easily performed that results in rapid elucidations of oncogene signatures, most essential genes, and drug sensitivity signatures. Our database contains dozens of tables and many of these table have 10 or more columns and millions of rows! This is a lot of data. And a lot of data is exactly what computational biologists and computer scientists with expertise in machine learning and artificial intelligence require to make predictions based on complex data sets.

I once heard a definition of machine learning/artificial intelligence that distinguishes it from classical computer science. It goes something like this. In classic computer science, a data set is entered into a computer. The computer *program* is essentially a set of rules about how to analyze the data. Thus, data are entered, analyzed by the rules, and the program provides a result. In Artificial Intelligence/machine learning, a data set is provided but here the answer is also provided, and the machine then develops the set of rules that connect the data with the answer. Thus, AI/ML is a method by which a machine analyzes data and *recognizes* what the data are describing. This type of analysis is perfect if one would like to use lots of data like the functional genomic data that we have (the data set) and link it to the drug sensitivity data that we also have (the answer) and develop a set of rules that allow the machine to recognize cells that are sensitive to a drug from those that are resistant.

We set out to test this idea using functional genomic data for one of my favorite drugs, Navitoclax. As described earlier, this drug targets the survival proteins coded for by the genes BCL2 and BCL2L1. We will see in the next chapter how identifying cells that are sensitive to this drug allowed us to develop drug combinations that acted synergistically to induce cancer cell-specific lethality. Thus, being able to predict sensitivity to Navitoclax in patients could be clinically useful. To illustrate this point further, Figure 10.1 shows the range of sensitivities to Navitoclax for the hundreds of cancer cell lines present in the Genomics of Drug Sensitivity in Cancer database. It can be seen from the figure that there is a 10,000-fold range in IC50s to this drug across the cell line panel. If one scans the GDSC database, it becomes obvious that this type of variation in drug sensitivity is the rule, not the exception, for many targeted cancer drugs. Thus, in the absence of any knowledge of the sensitivity of an individual patient to this drug, treatment with MTD doses will always be used resulting in fairly uniform off-target toxicity for all patients but with a wide range of effectiveness. Patients who are highly sensitive to the drug will have a good response and those with intermediate sensitivity or resistance will have a poor response or no response at all, and that won't be known until well into the course of therapy. Furthermore, for those patients with high drug sensitivity, it may have been possible for them to obtain great clinical benefit using a lower dose of the drug. Thus, if it could be predicted ahead of time which patients are sensitive to the drug and which are resistant, the drug could be used much more intelligently and with greater precision.

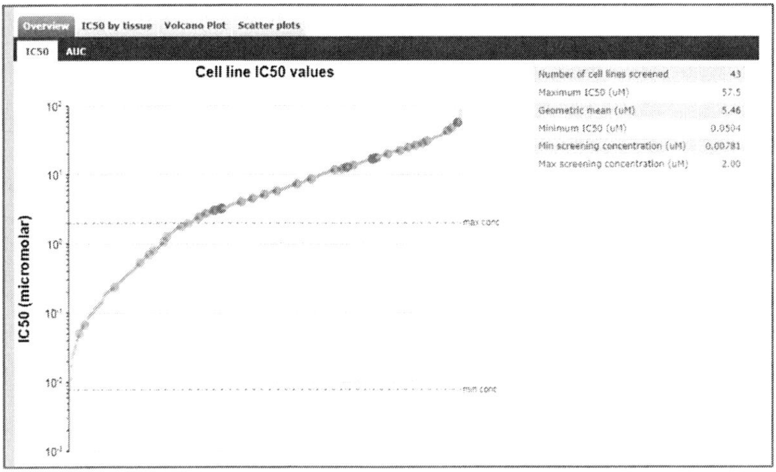

Figure 10.1. Range of sensitivities (IC50s) to Navitoclax for 967 cancer cell lines. The green and red dots show the IC50s for the 43 breast cancer cell lines tested. Note the log scale on the y-axis indicating a nearly 10,000-fold range in sensitivities to this drug for cancer cell lines. *See centrefold for this image in colour.*

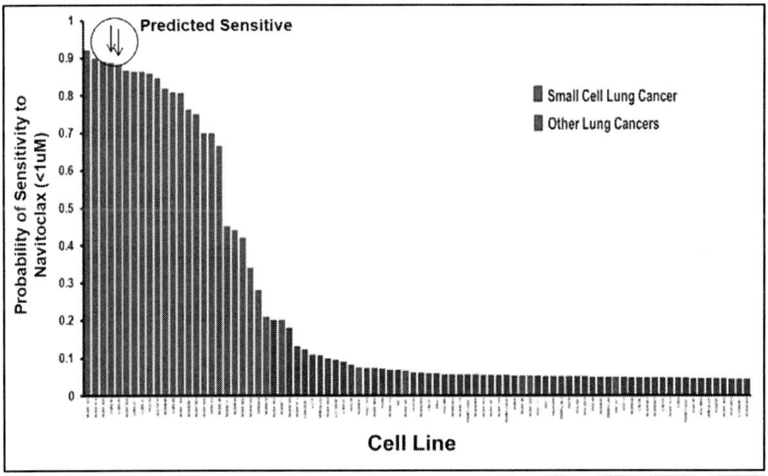

Figure 10.2. Distribution of probabilities of sensitivity to Navitoclax in 86 lung cancer cell lines. Red bars indicate small cell lung cancer lines and black bars indicate non-small cell lung cancer cell lines. *See centrefold for this image in colour.*

Okay so how can we do this, and can AI/ML provide some answers to this question? To test this idea, we downloaded the functional genomic data for 800 cancer cell lines (the data set) and the Navitoclax drug sensitivity data for those same cell lines from the genomics of drug sensitivity in cancer database (the answers). We then applied an AI/ML strategy to identify a signature of 20 genes that, based on their genomic status, predicted the probability that cells would be sensitive or resistance to Navitoclax. To test the predictive power of this algorithm, we obtained genomic data from 86 lung cancer cell lines for which Navitoclax sensitivity was not known and applied our algorithm. The one thing that was known about the cell line panel that we tested was that some were derived from small cell lung cancer, and some were derived from non-small cell lung cancer. Further, it was already known that, in general, small cell lung cancer cells are more sensitive to Navitoclax than non-small cell lung cancer cells.

The data in figure 10.2 shows that our AI/ML derived algorithm separated the small cell lung cancer cell lines from non-small cell lung cancer cell lines based on *predicted* Navitoclax sensitivity, which is consistent with what was already known about relative sensitivities to these two types of lung cancer. However, as can also be seen from the figure, the algorithm also predicted that some small cell lung cancer cell lines would be resistant to Navitoclax. To test this prediction, we obtained two small cell cancer cell lines that were predicted to be sensitive to Navitoclax and four of the small cell lung cancer cell lines that were predicted to be resistant to the drug and we determined the IC50s for Navitoclax on these six cell lines. The data in figure 10.3 shows that, indeed, three of the lines that were predicted to be resistant to Navitoclax were highly resistant and had IC50 doses orders of magnitude greater than those for the sensitive cell lines, despite the fact that the cells were derived from small cell lung cancer.

This is an exciting proof of concept that demonstrates that AI/ML methods can be used to train computers to *recognize* cells that are sensitive, intermediately sensitive, or resistant to individual targeted drugs. Once the AI/ML methods are established based on analysis of these types of very large data sets, individual unknown samples can be analyzed. All that is required is genomic data and gene expression data from the (patient) sample, and the algorithm can determine the probability that the individual sample will be drug sensitive. In other words, the algorithm determines how much an individual sample "looks like" sensitive or resistant cells.

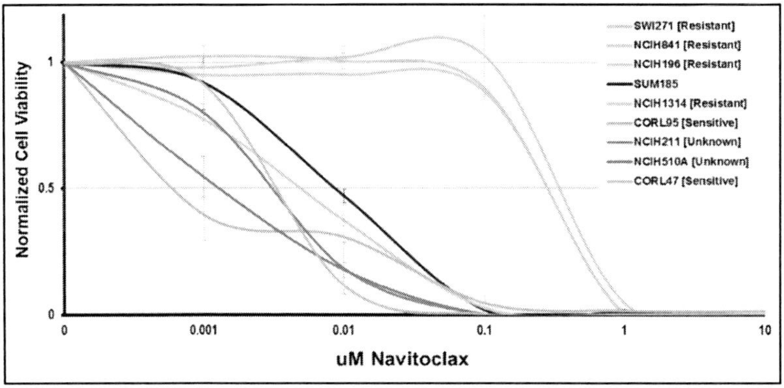

Figure 10.3. IC50 values for nine cancer cell lines treated with Navitoclax. Green lines were derived from small cell lung cancer cell lines that were predicted to be resistant to Navitoclax. *See centrefold for this image in colour.*

The work just described was our first attempt at applying AI/ML approaches to determine the potential for using large scale genomic data sets to predict sensitivity to a specific targeted drug. While highly encouraging, the strategy we employed is one of many potential AI/ML approaches that can be developed and tested to find the best strategy for using cancer cell line data to make accurate predictions about the sensitivity of an individual specimen to a range of targeted drugs.

In the example above, we used data for one drug across hundreds of cell lines to develop a predictive signature for sensitivity to the targeted drug. Clearly, this same approach can be extended to any number of targeted drugs, particularly those that are already FDA approved for clinical use, and in that way, improve our ability to use these drugs to impact patients.

There is, however, another strategy that also seeks to apply AI/ML methods that can predict the Tier 1, Tier 2, and Tier 3 drug sensitivity signatures described earlier, and in that way generate predictions for multiple drugs all at once. In this alternative approach, the AI/ML algorithm would use genomic data from a test specimen and computationally cluster that specimen to one or more cell lines in the database for which all gene essentialities and drug sensitivities are known. Such an approach would provide a quantitative value for "closeness" to one or more cell lines that could be used to make drug sensitivity predictions.

As an example of how such an approach might work, recall the data that was shown in figure 7.1 regarding the relationship between gene essentiality and drug sensitivity for breast cancer cell lines that overexpress the ESR1 gene (ERα). Recall also, that the relationship between ESR1 overexpression and gene essentiality was very strong, but the relationship between essentiality and sensitivity to three ER-targeted drugs was less robust. Now, imagine a specimen obtained from a breast cancer patient in which the ERα levels were clearly elevated, and the patient therefore considered a candidate for hormonal therapy. By applying our clustering-based AI/ML methods, we should be able to determine which of the many ER-positive cell lines that the patient is most like. If it turns out that the patient's genomic status indicates that the patient's cells are most like MCF-7 cells, this will predict high sensitivity to Tamoxifen and all other ERα targeted drugs. But what if, despite the presence of ERα expression, the genomics of the patient specimen indicated a high quantitative similarity to the cell line HCC1419? This cell line is resistant to Tamoxifen but is sensitive to the SERD drugs Fulvestrant and GDC1080. This type of prediction could prove to be highly valuable to both patient and oncologist because sensitivity to a SERD type drug relative to a SERM type drug is informative of the deep biology of the patient's breast cancer. Or consider a case where the patient specimen clusters tightly with the EFM19 cell line. This line not only overexpresses ERα, but also has a common PIK3CA mutation. The drug sensitivity signature for this line shows that the cells are sensitive to GDC0810 and also Alpelisib. In addition, these cells are highly sensitive to two different drugs that target effectors of the apoptosis pathway. In a similar way, a patient specimen that clustered with CAMA1 would bring into play not only ER-targeted drugs, but also AR targeted drugs, since these cells overexpress AR and are sensitive to the AR-drug Bicalutamide.

As an example of an ER-negative patient specimen, imagine that genomic data resulted in the specimen clustering with cell lines like DU4475. Based on the presence of the BRAF mutation, which is rare in breast cancer, this clustering would predict for high sensitivity to BRAF targeted drugs, since in this case, there is a strong correlation between essentiality of BRAF and sensitivity to BRAF targeted drugs. However, the Tier 1, 2, and 3 drug sensitivity signatures for DU4475 also predicts high sensitivity to several BCL2L1 targeted drugs, and this prediction would not be obvious by looking only at the genomics of BCL2 family members. Furthermore, the Tier 2 and Tier 3 sensitivities for this cell line suggest a number of other targeted drugs to which the patient cells would be highly sensitive, and all these data could be considered in developing a targeted drug treatment plan for the patient.

It is important to emphasize that I am not suggesting that a treatment plan for any patient be based solely on the quantitative association between the genomic features of a patient specimen and a single cell line. For this reason, the work being undertaken now is geared toward expanding our functional genomics database to include data from hundreds of cancer cell lines, instead of the 40 or so that we currently have. Once that is accomplished, our AI/ML strategy will allow us to associate quantitatively a patient specimen with a group of cell lines and common drug sensitivity features among that group of lines could be used to strengthen the drug sensitivity predictions. Having made these associations that predict drug sensitivity, one could then apply the previously described strategy to look for signatures that also predict for sensitivity to the same drugs. This type of orthogonal approach would be likely to be highly predictive for drugs to which patients exhibit sensitivity (or resistance), and this then would allow for possible drug combinations to be developed and used. More on this possibility in the next chapter.

In summary, the very volume of genomic and functional genomic data that have now been amassed for many thousands of cancer patients and for many hundreds of cancer-derived cell lines opens the door for the use of AI/ML approaches to get us closer to the elusive goal of true precision medicine for cancer. As we have described above, AI/ML approaches require large volumes of data for the algorithms that are used to correctly "recognize" either the drug sensitivity features of the specimen, or the cell line *likeness* features of a given cancer specimen. And it is the ability of these algorithms to recognize complex patters that emerge from complex data sets that makes this type of strategy ideally suited for improving precision medicine. But for this to happen, as I have argued throughout this book, we must take seriously the cell line data we have and recognize the power that these data sets have towards our goal of precision medicine for cancer. Because the ability to merge genomic features of candidate oncogenes with gene essentiality data and with drug sensitivity data is unique to cancer-derived cell lines. To ignore or diminish the importance of these data sets because of outmoded biases about cancer cell lines would be beyond unfortunate.

CHAPTER 11

USING FUNCTIONAL GENOMICS AND DRUG SENSITIVITY DATA TO PREDICT SYNERGISTIC DRUG COMBINATIONS IN BREAST CANCER CELL LINES

As a result of the now decades long development of various types of targeted drugs for cancer, the feature that determines how patients will respond is their sensitivity to these drugs. When patients exhibit sensitivity to a targeted drug, they experience clinical benefit with minimal, or easily manageable toxicity. By contrast, when patients respond poorly to a targeted drug, despite the presence of the biomarker that sometimes predicts sensitivity, they do not experience clinical benefit, though they do experience the toxic side effects to the drug. This is particularly true when, in an attempt to derive some level of clinical benefit, the drugs are used at their maximal tolerated doses (MTDs). Thus, if we can develop a strategy that, instead of measuring a single biomarker associated with a drug (e.g. expression of the estrogen receptor), integrates all of the functional genomic data to make a more precise prediction about targeted drug sensitivity, we could accomplish a paradigm shift that would move us away from using the of drugs at their maximum tolerated doses toward the use of drugs at their minimally effective doses (MEDs). This approach, if it can be achieved, offers the possibility of high levels of efficacy with minimal toxicity by using truly personalized and precise drug strategies for patients.

We have seen in the preceding chapters that sensitivity to targeted drugs that are in use in patients, particularly those that are tied to specific oncogenic events such as ERBB2 amplification, ESR1 overexpression, PIK3CA and BRAF mutations, are consistently observed in breast cancer cell lines with those same genomic alterations. Thus, as I have argued throughout this book, cancer cell lines are good reflections of the disease experienced by the patients from which the cell lines were derived.

There is another aspect of targeted drug sensitivity in cancer cells that has, heretofore, received relatively little attention in the scientific literature and even less attention in the clinical realm. That aspect has to do with our abilities to combine different targeted drugs. Targeted drug combinations offer the possibility of dramatically enhancing the therapeutic response experienced by a patient, either via additive effects of two different drugs, or via synergistic interactions that can occur with the use of specific drug combinations.

It is true that the idea of using combinations of targeted drugs in patients has been around for many years, and indeed, chemotherapeutic drugs are commonly administered in combinations. The main reason why targeted drug combinations haven't generated as much traction is because of the valid concern about toxicities being increased when more than one targeted drug is used. Once again, if two drugs are used at their maximum tolerated doses, off target toxicities are increased as well. I will argue that this concern can be overcome by correctly understanding the factors that influence drug sensitivities.

The traditional way of thinking about chemotherapy for cancer is that, if some amount of drug is good, more drug must be better. It is this thinking that underlies the design of phase I clinical trials for just about every type of cancer drug, the goal of which is to determine the maximum tolerated dose in patients for any given drug. And, while this approach has been effective for the development of chemotherapeutic drugs, it is not effective if one is considering combining targeted drugs, in which toxicities are likely to be amplified. Rather, the guiding principle for the combination of two or more targeted drugs should not be the maximum tolerated dose of each drug, but rather the minimally effective dose for each drug. That is, the lowest dose of a drug that gives maximum effect. As we have seen in our previous discussion about targeted drug sensitivities, whether presented as IC50 doses or Z-scores, the sensitivities for many drugs across a large panel of cell lines can vary by orders of magnitude. Thus, for a cell line (or patient) with high sensitivity to a given drug, a dose of 1 μM could be highly effective and essentially eradicate the growth or survival potential of the cells. By contrast, for cell lines (or patients) that exhibit less intrinsic sensitivity to the same drug, a dose of 1 μM might be only partially effective, or completely ineffective. However, that dose will carry similar side effects in all patients since most side effects are related to off-target effects of the drugs. Now, for those patients who are not particularly sensitive to a particular drug, increasing the dose to 10 μM or

100 μM will result in corresponding increases in response, and with increasing toxicities until one achieves the MTD for that particular drug.

Given that, if one truly wants to devise combinatorial targeted drug strategies that will have profound effects on growth/survival of cancer cells in the absence of significant toxicities, it will be essential to use drugs in cell lines or patients where the sensitivity to each drug is known so that appropriate doses can be used. Thus, in this strategy, one would strive to combine drugs at their minimally effective concentrations, and in this way achieve enhanced control of cancer cell growth and survival without undo toxicities.

As we have shown in our recent paper (Guest et al. 2016), this is not just a theoretical construct. During the development and characterization of the SUM Breast Cancer Cell Lines, we determined the oncogene signatures for each cell line and identified the essential genes in each line using an shRNA-based gene essentiality (drop-out) screen. Based on those results, we identified the oncogenes and other essential genes that are druggable and then initiated studies using drugs that target those functional oncogenes and other essential genes.

From these results, the SUM-185 cell line became particularly interesting because this cell line has three functional-druggable oncogenes: FGRR3, which is amplified and overexpressed, BCL2L1, which is also amplified and overexpressed, and PIK3CA which has a common point mutation. We then determined the sensitivity of this cell line to the three cognate targeted drugs, PD174071, Navitoclax, and A66 (similar to Alpelisib). Not surprisingly, we found SUM-185 cells to be highly sensitive to all three drugs.

Because the cells were so sensitive to all three targeted drugs, we then investigated the effectiveness of combining these drugs in two-drug or three-drug combinations. In these experiments, we were able to use low concentrations of each drug because of the exquisite sensitivity of the cells to each drug. The results of these experiments were striking and demonstrated that because of their sensitivity to low doses of the individual drugs, the combination of the FGFR targeted drug with Navitoclax resulted in synergistic cell lethality, and the three-drug combination enhanced that response by another order of magnitude. Overall, we found that a single administration of the three-drug combination reduced the clonogenic potential of SUM-185 cells by over 500-fold! And, because the sensitivity of the cells was such that we could use very low doses of each drug, combining the same three drugs in the same concentrations to other breast cancer cells that did not have the same genomic alterations, or to the normal breast epithelial cell line MCF-10A, did not result in any measurable decrease in clonogenic potential. Thus, by identifying druggable targets and drugs to which the cells are highly sensitive, we were able to achieve profound cancer cell lethality at doses that had no measurable effect on normal cells. Using this approach, we effectively reverse engineered SUM-185 cells. In subsequent experiments, we were able to use this same drug combination to induce dramatic regression of well-established SUM-185 xenograft tumors in SCID mise.

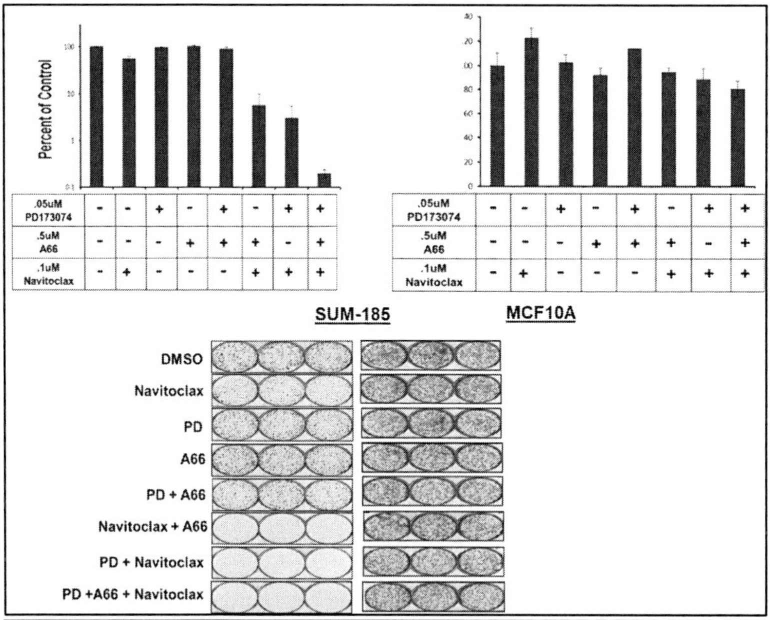

Figure 11.1. Effect of two and three targeted drug combinations on the clonogenic potential of SUM-185 breast cancer cells. Note the log scale of the left panel and the linear scale on the right panel showing profound induction of cancer cell lethality in the absence of any measurable loss of clonogenic potential of MCF-10A cells.

In the experiments described above using SUM-185 cells, we found there to be synergistic interactions between Navitoclax and either of the drugs that target the FGFR3 or PIK3CA. By contrast, there was no interaction when we combined the drug that targets FGFR3 and PIK3CA, which is not surprising since these oncogenes activate overlapping signaling pathways. This result points to potentially important interactions that involve oncogenes that drive cell proliferation, such as FGFR3 and PIK3CA, and those that promote cell survival, such as BCL2L1. Before going into this further, it is important at this point to emphasize a particular feature of how drug sensitivity experiments are performed that could be highly relevant to translation of these drug sensitivity studies to patients receiving these types of drugs.

When IC50 doses for individual targeted drugs are determined, they are typically arrived at using short-term proliferation assays. In such experiments, cells are exposed to a single application of a wide range of doses of the targeted drug of interest and cell number (usually indirectly measured!) is determined 72 hours after treatment. In these types of assays, it is difficult if not impossible to determine if the measured effect of the drug is based on the effect on the proliferation of the cells, or their loss of viability, since "cell number" is measured relative to non-treated cells that proliferate during the 72-hour incubation period. We wanted to investigate this further because, as important as drug sensitivity is to the understanding of drug-target interactions in cancer cells in the lab, in patients, what matters most is the ability of drugs to actually kill cancer cells.

Thus, in the experiments described above, we first determined the IC-50s for the three targeted drugs using traditional 72-hour proliferation assays and, indeed, found the cells to be highly sensitive to the oncogene-targeted drugs. However, when we performed the experiment in a different way, we obtained different results. One of the best, and time-tested ways of determining the effects of a drug on the *viability* of cancer cells is to perform clonogenic survival assays. In such experiments, cells are seeded at clonal densities and treated with varying concentrations of drugs for 72 hours. Then, the drug is washed out and the cells are allowed to proliferate and form colonies, or not, over a 10 day to two-week period. The idea is that if the growth inhibition that is observed in the 72-hour assays represents irreversible cell death or clonogenic death, this will be detected as a profound loss of clonogenic potential because for a clonogenic cell to give rise to a colony consisting of greater than 50 cells, that cell and its progeny must undergo approximately six population doublings. By contrast, if the reduction in cell numbers measured after just 72 hours is the result of an inhibition of proliferation that is reversible, then after washout of the drug, those cells will still give rise to colonies, albeit slightly smaller ones, or ones that take a bit longer to achieve the same number of cells per colony.

We wanted to determine which mechanism was operative in our experiments with targeted drugs in SUM-185 cells. We found that for both the FGFR inhibitor and the PIK3CA inhibitor, while highly effective at inhibiting *proliferation*, the drugs had little or no effect on the clonogenic potential of the cells following drug washout. Thus, even though the cells are highly sensitive to the drugs, the growth inhibition observed was almost completely *reversible*! By contrast, treatment of the cells with a low dose of Navitoclax reduced the clonogenic potential of the cells by about 50%, which isn't surprising since the BCL2L1 inhibitor interferes with cell survival pathways and not proliferation.

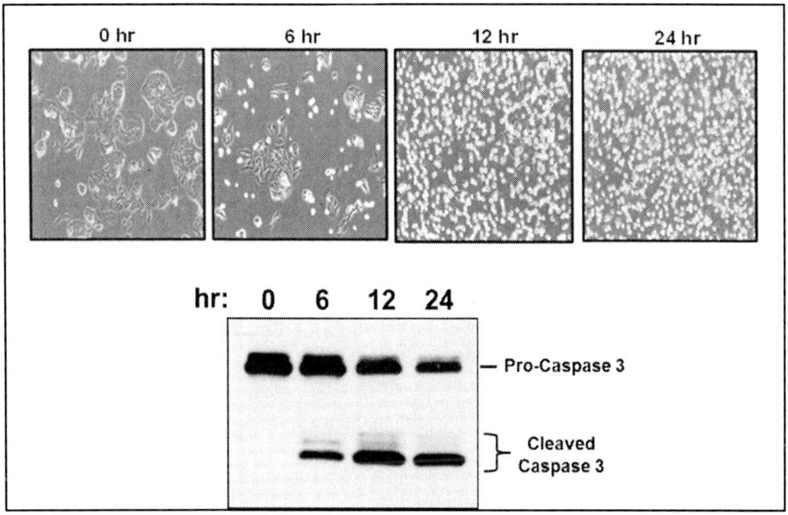

Figure 11.2. Induction of apoptosis (programmed cell death) in SUM-185 cells within 24 hours of exposure to low doses of Navitoclax and PD174074. Dead cells rounded up and detached from the ditch and the induction of cleaved Caspase 3 confirms the apoptotic mechanism of cell death.

Then, we examined the influence of the combined treatment of Navitoclax with either the FGFR or PIK3CA inhibitor using the clonogenic potential assay. In this version of the experiment, we found profound synergy in the ability of the drug combinations to induce irreversible clonogenic cell death. Thus, the excitement of this result is not only in the synergistic interaction of Navitoclax with two oncogene-targeted drugs, but that this synergy was directly related to the ability of these drugs to induce a profound and highly oncogene specific cell death.

Based on these results, we set out to explore the ability of Navitoclax to synergize with other oncogene targeted drugs in the SUM cell lines using an assay that is specifically designed to measure the presence of viable cells and to determine computationally the index of synergy between the two drugs in each cell line. The results of these experiments were consistent with the results using SUM-185 cells in several other cell lines and demonstrated that blocking cell survival pathways in combination with cell proliferation pathways can yield profound synergies with respect to cell viability. In other experiments, we found that a drug that targets PLK1 could act synergistically in combination with taxanes in triple negative breast cancer cells (Giordano et al. 2019).

These results highlight the potential for developing combinatorial targeted drug strategies that hinge on the ability to identify the drugs to which cells are highly sensitive. Further, these studies demonstrate the potential for synergy when simultaneously attacking essential targets in pathways that drive cell proliferation combined with attacking genes in pathways mediate cell survival, such as BCL2L1.

CHAPTER 12

REALITY CHECK

If there is one thing that we have learned in the past three decades during which we have strived to link mechanistic and causal aspects of cancer biology to the development of novel drugs and their incorporation into routine clinical use, is that making these leaps for even one drug against one target is a monumental task that requires years and millions (billions?) of dollars. There are a lot of good reasons for this, not the least of which is the necessity to demonstrate clinical safety and efficacy of any new drug that is developed for cancer. Indeed, the daunting level of this challenge has caused many a drug company to walk away from the enterprise altogether. And it is precisely because of the tried-and-true nature of cancer drug development methods that we ultimately group patients together based on single biomarkers associated with specific drugs all the while knowing that the predictive power of single biomarkers for drug efficacy is not very good. Otherwise, how else are we to do clinical trials of novel drugs? Grouping patients is necessary to have sufficient numbers to provide statistical power to results of these clinical trials because without that, no drugs would leave the pipeline and enter the clinic.

And yet, in this book, I am advocating for an entirely different approach for the development of precision medicine strategies for individual patients with cancer. And I argue that we need new and novel approaches because, as I've said now many times, there is still no cure for metastatic disease. The conventional methods, while being highly successful for achieving local control of cancer and delaying or preventing recurrence and metastatic spread, have largely failed for patients who develop overt metastatic disease. That said, how on earth can we ever perform the clinical studies, not to mention further pre-clinical studies, that would be necessary to validate this approach for use in patients with metastatic disease? What I am advocating here is nothing less than a sea change in how we evaluate cancer patients in developing treatment plans, and to say that this won't be easy would be a vast understatement. But a sea change seems to be necessary.

Given that, I will end this monograph with two proposals for strategies that could allow us to move this approach forward, assuming that we are successful in developing the Artificial Intelligence/Machine Learning strategies that make sensitivity predictions for FDA-approved targeted drugs as well as other drugs in the developmental pipeline.

The first approach involves collaboration with groups of investigators that have developed both PDX and organoid models of cancer. There are literally hundreds of such models that have now been developed for many cancer types and obtaining genomic data from any or all of them using currently available methods would be straight forward, and essentially the same as what we might eventually do with patient samples. The goals of the groups who have developed these PDX and organoid models has always been to use them to test specific drugs and drug combinations. Thus, I propose a merger, if you will, between the cell line-oriented groups and the PDX/organoid groups to test the predictions made by our AI/ML methods. While we will be well positioned to use genomic data obtained from these models to make predictions about drug strategies based on predicted drug sensitivity, our collaborators are well positioned to test these predictions in their models. Thus, this type of interaction offers the possibility of testing and validating predictions made using cell line data in model systems that some consider to be better, or at least closer to the human disease, than the cell lines. Obviously, I predict that the drug sensitivity predictions that will emerge from our analysis of genomic data derived from these other model types will be borne out, which would provide the next level of preclinical data needed to advance the drug prediction strategy to clinical studies.

The second approach is actually not as difficult as one might imagine because as a field, we have already embarked on just the type of trial that could be used to test AI/ML based drug sensitivity predictions. The NCI-MATCH trial was designed to be a nationwide basket trial in which patients were placed into baskets not because of the type of cancer they have, but because of the type of genomic alterations present in their cancers (Flaherty, Gray, Chen, Li, Patton, et al. 2020; Flaherty, Gray, Chen, Li, McShane, et al. 2020; "NCI-MATCH Sets "Benchmark of Actionability"" 2021; Murciano-Goroff, Drilon, and Stadler 2021). And then, once assigned to a particular basket, patients were treated on the clinical trial using targeted drugs associated with their particular genomic feature. This has been a highly innovative trial the results of which have been somewhat disappointing because as we have learned from this trial, not to mention other findings from other trials, a single biomarker or genomic feature by itself is not a very strong predictor of targeted drug sensitivity. And alas, this is exactly what would have been predicted based on analysis of cell line data, as was shown in chapter 7. Given that, if we are able to use AI/ML strategies derived from cell line data to develop drug sensitivity signatures and use these signatures instead of single biomarkers, the same design developed for the NCI-MATCH trial could be used. In this version of the MATCH trial, patients would be assigned to their drug baskets based on predicted drug sensitivities that were derived from the full complement of functional genomics data instead of a single biomarker. Alternatively, it may be possible to re-interpret current data based on an AI/ML analysis of the genomic data already obtained from patients on the trial. Since it will be straight forward to run the AI/ML algorithms using the same types of genomic data already being collected for the NCI-MATCH trial, the overall infrastructure for conducting the trial could be used again. Thus, this future version of MATCH would be well suited for the ultimate clinical test of drug sensitivity algorithms to develop targeted drug treatment plans for patients.

There is no cure for metastatic disease

Over the past few years, the following phrase has come to be used in a number of social and scientific situations: "the definition of insanity is the repeated applications of the same failed strategy and hoping for a different result", or something like that. When it comes to treating metastatic disease, we really do try the same failed strategies over and over again, while treating oncologists know, all too well, the outcome. It's time for us to try something different. For patients with metastatic disease, it is becoming more and more common to biopsy metastatic lesions, which can be sequenced to provide genomic data for individual metastatic lesions. It is our goal, one day, to use genomic data from metastatic lesions to make better predictions about the drugs to which a patient will be sensitive, or resistant, and do that in a way that will allow for rational and safe drug combinations to be tried. At some point, we have to get more creative in how we treat patients with metastatic disease who have often already failed conventional therapy. Because otherwise, the phrase "there is no cure for metastatic disease" will continue to be true, and we have come too far to be satisfied with that.

REFERENCES

Agrawal, A., E. Gutteridge, J. M. Gee, R. I. Nicholson, and J. F. Robertson. 2005. "Overview of tyrosine kinase inhibitors in clinical breast cancer." *Endocrine-related cancer* 12 Suppl 1: S135-44. https://doi.org/10.1677/erc.1.01059. http://www.ncbi.nlm.nih.gov/pubmed/16113090.

Andre, F., T. Bachelot, M. Campone, F. Dalenc, J. M. Perez-Garcia, S. A. Hurvitz, N. Turner, H. Rugo, J. W. Smith, S. Deudon, M. Shi, Y. Zhang, A. Kay, D. G. Porta, A. Yovine, and J. Baselga. 2013. "Targeting FGFR with dovitinib (TKI258): preclinical and clinical data in breast cancer." *Clin Cancer Res* 19 (13): 3693-702. https://doi.org/10.1158/1078-0432.CCR-13-0190. https://www.ncbi.nlm.nih.gov/pubmed/23658459.

Angrand, P. O., F. Apiou, A. F. Stewart, B. Dutrillaux, R. Losson, and P. Chambon. 2001. "NSD3, a new SET domain-containing gene, maps to 8p12 and is amplified in human breast cancer cell lines." *Genomics* 74 (1): 79-88. http://www.ncbi.nlm.nih.gov/entrez/query.fcgi?cmd=Retrieve&db=PubMed&dopt=Citation&list_uids=11374904.

Armaghani, A. J., and H. S. Han. 2020. "Alpelisib in the Treatment of Breast Cancer: A Short Review on the Emerging Clinical Data." *Breast Cancer (Dove Med Press)* 12: 251-258. https://doi.org/10.2147/BCTT.S219436. https://www.ncbi.nlm.nih.gov/pubmed/33239910.

Bargmann, C.I., M.C. Hung, and R.A. Weinberg. 1986. "Multiple independent activations of the c-neu oncogene by a point mutation altering the trans-membrane domain of p185." *Cell* 45: 649-657.

Bautista, S., and C. Theillet. 1998. "CCND1 and FGFR1 coamplification results in the colocalization of 11q13 and 8p12 sequences in breast tumor nuclei." *Genes Chromosomes Cancer* 22 (4): 268-277.

Behbod, F., F. S. Kittrell, H. LaMarca, D. Edwards, S. Kerbawy, J. C. Heestand, E. Young, P. Mukhopadhyay, H. W. Yeh, D. C. Allred, M. Hu, K. Polyak, J. M. Rosen, and D. Medina. 2009. "An intraductal human-in-mouse transplantation model mimics the subtypes of ductal carcinoma in situ." *Breast Cancer Res* 11 (5): R66. https://doi.org/10.1186/bcr2358. https://www.ncbi.nlm.nih.gov/pubmed/19735549.

Berns, E.M.J.J., J.A. Foekens, W.L.J. van Putten, I.L. van Stavern, H. Portengen, W.C.H. De Koning, and J.G.M. Klijn. 1992. "Prognostic factors in human primary breast cancer: Compairosn of *c-myc* and HER*2/neu* amplification." *J Steroid Biochem Mol Biol* 43 (1-3): 13-19.

Beroukhim, R., C. H. Mermel, D. Porter, G. Wei, S. Raychaudhuri, J. Donovan, J. Barretina, J. S. Boehm, J. Dobson, M. Urashima, K. T. Mc Henry, R. M. Pinchback, A. H. Ligon, Y. J. Cho, L. Haery, H. Greulich, M. Reich, W. Winckler, M. S. Lawrence, B. A. Weir, K. E. Tanaka, D. Y. Chiang, A. J. Bass, A. Loo, C. Hoffman, J. Prensner, T. Liefeld, Q. Gao, D. Yecies, S. Signoretti, E. Maher, F. J. Kaye, H. Sasaki, J. E. Tepper, J. A. Fletcher, J. Tabernero, J. Baselga, M. S. Tsao, F. Demichelis, M. A. Rubin, P. A. Janne, M. J. Daly, C. Nucera, R. L. Levine, B. L. Ebert, S. Gabriel, A. K. Rustgi, C. R. Antonescu, M. Ladanyi, A. Letai, L. A. Garraway, M. Loda, D. G. Beer, L. D. True, A. Okamoto, S. L. Pomeroy, S. Singer, T. R. Golub, E. S. Lander, G. Getz, W. R. Sellers, and M. Meyerson. 2010. "The landscape of somatic copy-number alteration across human cancers." *Nature* 463 (7283): 899-905. https://doi.org/10.1038/nature08822. http://www.ncbi.nlm.nih.gov/pubmed/20164920.

Borg, A., B. Baldetorp, M. Ferno, D. Killander, H. Olsson, and H. Sigurdsson. 1991. "ERBB2 Amplification in Breast Cancer with a High Rate of Proliferation." *Oncogene* 6 (1): 137-143.

Brady, N., P. Chuntova, L. K. Bade, and K. L. Schwertfeger. 2013. "The FGF/FGFR axis as a therapeutic target in breast cancer." *Expert Rev Endocrinol Metab* 8 (4): 391-402. https://doi.org/10.1586/17446651.2013.811910. https://www.ncbi.nlm.nih.gov/pubmed/25400686.

Brown, M. S., B. Abdollahi, O. M. Wilkins, H. Lu, P. Chakraborty, N. B. Ognjenovic, K. E. Muller, M. K. Jolly, B. C. Christensen, S. Hassanpour, and D. R. Pattabiraman. 2022. "Phenotypic heterogeneity driven by plasticity of the intermediate EMT state governs disease progression and metastasis in breast cancer." *Sci Adv* 8 (31): eabj8002. https://doi.org/10.1126/sciadv.abj8002. https://www.ncbi.nlm.nih.gov/pubmed/35921406.

Carlson, J. J., and J. A. Roth. 2013. "The impact of the Oncotype Dx breast cancer assay in clinical practice: a systematic review and meta-analysis." *Breast Cancer Res Treat* 141 (1): 13-22. https://doi.org/10.1007/s10549-013-2666-z. https://www.ncbi.nlm.nih.gov/pubmed/23974828.

Charafe-Jauffret, E., C. Ginestier, F. Iovino, J. Wicinski, N. Cervera, P. Finetti, M. H. Hur, M. E. Diebel, F. Monville, J. Dutcher, M. Brown,

P. Viens, L. Xerri, F. Bertucci, G. Stassi, G. Dontu, D. Birnbaum, and M. S. Wicha. 2009. "Breast cancer cell lines contain functional cancer stem cells with metastatic capacity and a distinct molecular signature." *Cancer Res* 69 (4): 1302-13. http://www.ncbi.nlm.nih.gov/entrez/query.fcgi?cmd=Retrieve&db=PubMed&dopt=Citation&list_uids=19190339

Cobleigh, M., C. Vogel, D. Tripathy, N. Robert, S. Scholl, L. Fehrenbacher, V. Paton, S. Shak, G. Lieberman, and D. Slamon. 1998. "Efficacy and safety of Herceptin (humanized anti-HER2 antibody) as a single agent in 222 women with HER2 overexpression who relapsed following chemotherapy for metastatic breast cancer." *Proc of ASCO* 376 (17): 97A.

Cohen, J.B., and A.D. Levinson. 1988. "A point mutation in the last intron responsible for increased expression and transforming activity of the c-Has-ras oncogene #226." *Nature* 334: 119-124.

Collins, F. S. 1997. "Sequencing the human genome." *Hosp Pract (1995)* 32 (1): 35-43, 46-9, 53-4. https://doi.org/10.1080/21548331.1997.11443403. https://www.ncbi.nlm.nih.gov/pubmed/9006582.

Coppola, Domenico. 2010. *Mechanisms of Oncogenesis*. Vol. 12. Springer.

Copur, M. S. 2020. "Alpelisib to treat breast cancer." *Drugs Today (Barc)* 56 (6): 357-363. https://doi.org/10.1358/dot.2020.56.6.3137526. https://www.ncbi.nlm.nih.gov/pubmed/32525134.

Cory, S. 1986. "Activation of cellular oncogenes in hemopoietic cells by chromosome translocation." *Adv Cancer Res* 47: 189-234. https://doi.org/10.1016/s0065-230x(08)60200-6. https://www.ncbi.nlm.nih.gov/pubmed/3096089.

Cucciniello, L., L. Gerratana, L. Del Mastro, and F. Puglisi. 2022. "Tailoring adjuvant endocrine therapy in early breast cancer: When, how, and how long?" *Cancer Treat Rev* 110: 102445. https://doi.org/10.1016/j.ctrv.2022.102445. https://www.ncbi.nlm.nih.gov/pubmed/35944419.

Curtit, E., L. Mansi, Y. Maisonnette-Escot, J. L. Sautiere, and X. Pivot. 2017. "Prognostic and predictive indicators in early-stage breast cancer and the role of genomic profiling: Focus on the Oncotype DX((R)) Breast Recurrence Score Assay." *Eur J Surg Oncol* 43 (5): 921-930. https://doi.org/10.1016/j.ejso.2016.11.016. https://www.ncbi.nlm.nih.gov/pubmed/28087099.

David Jenkins, F. Xavier Bosch. 2019. *Human Papillomavirus*. Academic Press.

De Luca, A., D. Frezzetti, M. Gallo, and N. Normanno. 2017. "FGFR-targeted therapeutics for the treatment of breast cancer." *Expert Opin Investig Drugs* 26 (3): 303-311. https://doi.org/10.1080/13543784.2017.1287173. https://www.ncbi.nlm.nih.gov/pubmed/28121208.

Deininger, M. W., and B. J. Druker. 2003. "Specific targeted therapy of chronic myelogenous leukemia with imatinib." *Pharmacol Rev* 55 (3): 401-23. https://doi.org/10.1124/pr.55.3.4. http://www.ncbi.nlm.nih.gov/pubmed/12869662.

Dickson, R. B., and M. M. Gottesman. 1990. "Understanding of the molecular basis of drug resistance in cancer reveals new targets for chemotherapy." *Trends Pharmacol Sci* 11 (8): 305-7. https://doi.org/10.1016/0165-6147(90)90227-y. https://www.ncbi.nlm.nih.gov/pubmed/2203190.

Dontu, G., W. M. Abdallah, J. M. Foley, K. W. Jackson, M. F. Clarke, M. J. Kawamura, and M. S. Wicha. 2003. "In vitro propagation and transcriptional profiling of human mammary stem/progenitor cells." *Genes Dev* 17 (10): 1253-70. http://www.ncbi.nlm.nih.gov/entrez/query.fcgi?cmd=Retrieve&db=PubMed&dopt=Citation&list_uids=12756227

Druker, B. J. 2008. "Translation of the Philadelphia chromosome into therapy for CML." *Blood* 112 (13): 4808-17. https://doi.org/10.1182/blood-2008-07-077958. http://www.ncbi.nlm.nih.gov/pubmed/19064740.

Druker, B. J., C. L. Sawyers, H. Kantarjian, D. J. Resta, S. F. Reese, J. M. Ford, R. Capdeville, and M. Talpaz. 2001. "Activity of a specific inhibitor of the BCR-ABL tyrosine kinase in the blast crisis of chronic myeloid leukemia and acute lymphoblastic leukemia with the Philadelphia chromosome." *N Engl J Med* 344 (14): 1038-42. https://doi.org/10.1056/NEJM200104053441402. http://www.ncbi.nlm.nih.gov/pubmed/11287973.

Druker, BJ, M Talpaz, DJ Resta, B Peng, E Buchdunger, JM Ford, NB Lydon, H Kantarjian, R Capdeville, S Ohno-Jones, and CL Sawyers. 2001. "Efficacy and safety of a specific inhibitor of the BCR-ABL tyrosine kinase in chronic myeloid leukemia." *N Engl J Med* 344 (14): 1031-7.

Druker, BJ, S Tamura, E Buchdunger, S Ohno, GM Segal, S Fanning, J Zimmermann, and NB Lydon. 1996. "Effects of a selective inhibitor of the Abl tyrosine kinase on the growth of Bcr-Abl positive cells." *Nat Med* 2 (5): 561-6.

Ethier, S.P. 1985. "Primary culture and serial passage of normal and carcinogen-treated rat mammary epithelial cells in vitro #6." *J Natl Cancer Inst* 74: 1307-1318.

—. 1986. "Serum-free culture conditions for the growth of normal rat mammary epithelial cells in primary culture." *In Vitro Cell Dev Biol* 22: 485-490.

Ethier, S.P., and K.C. Cundiff. 1987. "Importance of extended growth potential and growth factor independence on in vivo neoplastic potential of primary rat mammary carcinoma cells." *Cancer Res* 47 (20): 5316-5322.

Ethier, S.P., and R. Moorthy. 1991. "Multiple Growth Factor Independence in Rat Mammary Carcinoma Cells." *Breast Cancer Res Treat* 18 (2): 73-81.

Ethier, S.P., R.M. Summerfelt, K.C. Cundiff, and B.B. Asch. 1990. "The influence of growth factors on the proliferative potential of normal and primary breast cancer-derived human breast epithelial cells." *Breast Cancer Res Treat* 17: 221-230.

Fink, L., and F. S. Collins. 1997. "The Human Genome Project: view from the National Institutes of Health." *J Am Med Womens Assoc (1972)* 52 (1): 4-7, 15. https://www.ncbi.nlm.nih.gov/pubmed/9033164.

Flaherty, K. T., R. Gray, A. Chen, S. Li, D. Patton, S. R. Hamilton, P. M. Williams, E. P. Mitchell, A. J. Iafrate, J. Sklar, L. N. Harris, L. M. McShane, L. V. Rubinstein, D. J. Sims, M. Routbort, B. Coffey, T. Fu, J. A. Zwiebel, R. F. Little, D. Marinucci, R. Catalano, R. Magnan, W. Kibbe, C. Weil, J. V. Tricoli, B. Alexander, S. Kumar, G. K. Schwartz, F. Meric-Bernstam, C. J. Lih, W. McCaskill-Stevens, P. Caimi, N. Takebe, V. Datta, C. L. Arteaga, J. S. Abrams, R. Comis, P. J. O'Dwyer, B. A. Conley, and Nci-Match Team. 2020. "The Molecular Analysis for Therapy Choice (NCI-MATCH) Trial: Lessons for Genomic Trial Design." *J Natl Cancer Inst* 112 (10): 1021-1029. https://doi.org/10.1093/jnci/djz245. https://www.ncbi.nlm.nih.gov/pubmed/31922567.

Flaherty, K. T., R. J. Gray, A. P. Chen, S. Li, L. M. McShane, D. Patton, S. R. Hamilton, P. M. Williams, A. J. Iafrate, J. Sklar, E. P. Mitchell, L. N. Harris, N. Takebe, D. J. Sims, B. Coffey, T. Fu, M. Routbort, J. A. Zwiebel, L. V. Rubinstein, R. F. Little, C. L. Arteaga, R. Comis, J. S. Abrams, P. J. O'Dwyer, B. A. Conley, and Nci-Match team. 2020. "Molecular Landscape and Actionable Alterations in a Genomically Guided Cancer Clinical Trial: National Cancer Institute Molecular Analysis for Therapy Choice (NCI-MATCH)." *J Clin Oncol* 38 (33): 3883-3894. https://doi.org/10.1200/JCO.19.03010.

https://www.ncbi.nlm.nih.gov/pubmed/33048619.

Forozan, F., E.H. Mahlamaki, O. Monni, Y. Chen, R. Veldman, Y. Jiang, G. Gooden, S.P. Ethier, A. Kallioniemi, and O-P. Kallioniemi. 2000. "CGH analysis of 38 breast cancer cell lines: A basis for interpreting cDNA mircroarray data." *Cancer Res* 60: 4519-4525.

Forozan, F., R. Veldman, C.A. Ammerman, N.Z. Parsa, A. Kallioniemi, O. Kallioniemi, and S.P. Ethier. 1999. "Molecular cytogenetic analysis of 11 new human breast cancer cell lines." *Br J Cancer* 81 (8): 1328-1334.

Freedman, L. P., M. C. Gibson, S. P. Ethier, H. R. Soule, R. M. Neve, and Y. A. Reid. 2015. "Reproducibility: changing the policies and culture of cell line authentication." *Nat Methods* 12 (6): 493-7. https://doi.org/10.1038/nmeth.3403. https://www.ncbi.nlm.nih.gov/pubmed/26020501.

Freedman, L. P., M. C. Gibson, R. Wisman, S. P. Ethier, H. R. Soule, Y. A. Reid, and R. M. Neve. 2015. "The culture of cell culture practices and authentication--Results from a 2015 Survey." *Biotechniques* 59 (4): 189-90, 192. https://doi.org/10.2144/000114344. https://www.ncbi.nlm.nih.gov/pubmed/26458546.

Galvani, E., R. Alfieri, E. Giovannetti, A. Cavazzoni, S. La Monica, M. Galetti, C. Fumarola, M. Bonelli, M. Mor, M. Tiseo, G. J. Peters, P. G. Petronini, and A. Ardizzoni. 2013. "Epidermal growth factor receptor tyrosine kinase inhibitors: current status and future perspectives in the development of novel irreversible inhibitors for the treatment of mutant non-small cell lung cancer." *Current pharmaceutical design* 19 (5): 818-32. http://www.ncbi.nlm.nih.gov/pubmed/22973953.

Ginestier, C., M. H. Hur, E. Charafe-Jauffret, F. Monville, J. Dutcher, M. Brown, J. Jacquemier, P. Viens, C. G. Kleer, S. Liu, A. Schott, D. Hayes, D. Birnbaum, M. S. Wicha, and G. Dontu. 2007. "ALDH1 is a marker of normal and malignant human mammary stem cells and a predictor of poor clinical outcome." *Cell Stem Cell* 1 (5): 555-67. http://www.ncbi.nlm.nih.gov/entrez/query.fcgi?cmd=Retrieve&db=PubMed&dopt=Citation&list_uids=18371393

Giordano, A., Y. Liu, K. Armeson, Y. Park, M. Ridinger, M. Erlander, J. Reuben, C. Britten, C. Kappler, E. Yeh, and S. Ethier. 2019. "Polo-like kinase 1 (Plk1) inhibition synergizes with taxanes in triple negative breast cancer." *PLoS One* 14 (11): e0224420. https://doi.org/10.1371/journal.pone.0224420. https://www.ncbi.nlm.nih.gov/pubmed/31751384.

Goncalves, J. M., M. M. R. Cordeiro, and E. R. C. Rivero. 2017. "The Role of the Complex USP1/WDR48 in Differentiation and Proliferation

Processes in Cancer Stem Cells." *Curr Stem Cell Res Ther* 12 (5): 416-422. https://doi.org/10.2174/1574888X12666170315104013. https://www.ncbi.nlm.nih.gov/pubmed/28302046.

Gonen, M., B. A. Weir, G. S. Cowley, F. Vazquez, Y. Guan, A. Jaiswal, M. Karasuyama, V. Uzunangelov, T. Wang, A. Tsherniak, S. Howell, D. Marbach, B. Hoff, T. C. Norman, A. Airola, A. Bivol, K. Bunte, D. Carlin, S. Chopra, A. Deran, K. Ellrott, P. Gopalacharyulu, K. Graim, S. Kaski, S. A. Khan, Y. Newton, S. Ng, T. Pahikkala, E. Paull, A. Sokolov, H. Tang, J. Tang, K. Wennerberg, Y. Xie, X. Zhan, F. Zhu, Dream Community Broad, T. Aittokallio, H. Mamitsuka, J. M. Stuart, J. S. Boehm, D. E. Root, G. Xiao, G. Stolovitzky, W. C. Hahn, and A. A. Margolin. 2017. "A Community Challenge for Inferring Genetic Predictors of Gene Essentialities through Analysis of a Functional Screen of Cancer Cell Lines." *Cell Syst* 5 (5): 485-497 e3. https://doi.org/10.1016/j.cels.2017.09.004. https://www.ncbi.nlm.nih.gov/pubmed/28988802.

Groffen, J., and N. C. Heisterkamp. 1989. "Philadelphia chromosome translocation." *Crit Rev Oncog* 1 (1): 53-64. https://www.ncbi.nlm.nih.gov/pubmed/2488124.

Guest, S. T., Z. R. Kratche, A. Bollig-Fischer, R. Haddad, and S. P. Ethier. 2015. "Two members of the TRiC chaperonin complex, CCT2 and TCP1 are essential for survival of breast cancer cells and are linked to driving oncogenes." *Exp Cell Res* 332 (2): 223-35. https://doi.org/10.1016/j.yexcr.2015.02.005. http://www.ncbi.nlm.nih.gov/pubmed/25704758.

Guest, S. T., Z. R. Kratche, J. C. Irish, R. C. Wilson, R. Haddad, J. W. Gray, E. Garrett-Mayer, and S. P. Ethier. 2016. "Functional oncogene signatures guide rationally designed combination therapies to synergistically induce breast cancer cell death." *Oncotarget*. https://doi.org/10.18632/oncotarget.9147. http://www.ncbi.nlm.nih.gov/pubmed/27153554.

Guyer, M. S., and F. S. Collins. 1993. "The Human Genome Project and the future of medicine." *Am J Dis Child* 147 (11): 1145-52. https://doi.org/10.1001/archpedi.1993.02160350019003. https://www.ncbi.nlm.nih.gov/pubmed/8237907.

Haluska, F. G., and C. M. Croce. 1987. "Molecular mechanisms of chromosome translocation in human B- and T-cell neoplasia." *Ann N Y Acad Sci* 511: 196-206. https://doi.org/10.1111/j.1749-6632.1987.tb36248.x. https://www.ncbi.nlm.nih.gov/pubmed/3326464.

Haluska, F. G., Y. Tsujimoto, and C. M. Croce. 1987. "Oncogene activation by chromosome translocation in human malignancy." *Annu Rev Genet* 21: 321-45. https://doi.org/10.1146/annurev.ge.21.120187.001541. https://www.ncbi.nlm.nih.gov/pubmed/3327468.

Hammond, S.L., R.G. Ham, and M.R. Stampfer. 1984. "Serum-free growth of human mammary epithelial cells: rapid clonal growth in defined medium and extended serial passage with pituitary extract #58." *Proc Natl Acad Sci U S A* 81: 5435-5439.

Hanahan, D., and R. A. Weinberg. 2000. "The hallmarks of cancer." *Cell* 100 (1): 57-70. http://www.ncbi.nlm.nih.gov/pubmed/10647931.

—. 2011. "Hallmarks of cancer: the next generation." *Cell* 144 (5): 646-74. https://doi.org/10.1016/j.cell.2011.02.013. http://www.ncbi.nlm.nih.gov/pubmed/21376230.

Hatsukami, Stephen S. Hecht and Dorothhy K. 2022. *Tobacco And Cancer: The Science and the Story*. edited by Stephen S. Hecht and Dorothhy K. Hatsukami: World Scientific.

Heakal, Y., M. Kester, and S. Savage. 2011. "Vemurafenib (PLX4032): an orally available inhibitor of mutated BRAF for the treatment of metastatic melanoma." *Ann Pharmacother* 45 (11): 1399-405. https://doi.org/10.1345/aph.1Q363. https://www.ncbi.nlm.nih.gov/pubmed/22028422.

Heppner, G. H., D. L. Dexter, T. DeNucci, F. R. Miller, and P. Calabresi. 1978. "Heterogeneity in drug sensitivity among tumor cell subpopulations of a single mammary tumor." *Cancer Res* 38 (11 Pt 1): 3758-63. https://www.ncbi.nlm.nih.gov/pubmed/698935.

Heppner, G. H., S. E. Loveless, F. R. Miller, K. H. Mahoney, and A. M. Fulton. 1983. "Mammary tumor heterogeneity." *Symp Fundam Cancer Res* 36: 209-21. https://www.ncbi.nlm.nih.gov/pubmed/6382505.

Heppner, G., K. Yamashina, B. Miller, and F. Miller. 1986. "Tumor heterogeneity in metastasis." *Prog Clin Biol Res* 212: 45-59. https://www.ncbi.nlm.nih.gov/pubmed/3714732.

Hui, R., D.H. Campbell, C.S.L. Lee, K. McCaul, D.J. Horsfall, E.A. Musgrove, R.J. Daly, R. Seshadri, and R.L. Sutherland. 1997. "EMS1 amplification can occur independently of CCND1 or INT-2 amplification at 11q13 and may identify different phenotypes in primary breast cancer." *Oncogene* 15 (13): 1617-1623.

Irish, J. C., J. N. Mills, B. Turner-Ivey, R. C. Wilson, S. T. Guest, A. Rutkovsky, A. Dombkowski, C. S. Kappler, G. Hardiman, and S. P. Ethier. 2016. "Amplification of WHSC1L1 regulates expression and estrogen-independent activation of ERalpha in SUM-44 breast cancer cells and is associated with ERalpha over-expression in breast cancer." *Mol Oncol*. https://doi.org/10.1016/j.molonc.2016.02.003. http://www.ncbi.nlm.nih.gov/pubmed/27005559.

Jordan, E. J., and C. M. Kelly. 2012. "Vemurafenib for the treatment of melanoma." *Expert Opin Pharmacother* 13 (17): 2533-43. https://doi.org/10.1517/14656566.2012.737780. https://www.ncbi.nlm.nih.gov/pubmed/23094782.

Jordan, V. C. 2006. "Tamoxifen (ICI46,474) as a targeted therapy to treat and prevent breast cancer." *Br J Pharmacol* 147 Suppl 1: S269-76. https://doi.org/10.1038/sj.bjp.0706399. https://www.ncbi.nlm.nih.gov/pubmed/16402113.

—. 2008. "Tamoxifen: catalyst for the change to targeted therapy." *Eur J Cancer* 44 (1): 30-8. https://doi.org/10.1016/j.ejca.2007.11.002. https://www.ncbi.nlm.nih.gov/pubmed/18068350.

—. 2014. "Tamoxifen as the first targeted long-term adjuvant therapy for breast cancer." *Endocr Relat Cancer* 21 (3): R235-46. https://doi.org/10.1530/ERC-14-0092. https://www.ncbi.nlm.nih.gov/pubmed/24659478.

—. 2021. "50th anniversary of the first clinical trial with ICI 46,474 (tamoxifen): then what happened?" *Endocr Relat Cancer* 28 (1): R11-R30. https://doi.org/10.1530/ERC-20-0335. https://www.ncbi.nlm.nih.gov/pubmed/33151906.

Kallioniemi, O. P., A. Kallioniemi, W. Kurisu, A. Thor, L. C. Chen, H. S. Smith, F. M. Waldman, D. Pinkel, and J. W. Gray. 1992. "ERBB2 amplification in breast cancer analyzed by fluorescence in situ hybridization." *Proc Natl Acad Sci U S A* 89 (12): 5321-5. http://www.ncbi.nlm.nih.gov/entrez/query.fcgi?cmd=Retrieve&db=PubMed&dopt=Citation&list_uids=1351679.

Kim, S. Y., and W. C. Hahn. 2007. "Cancer genomics: integrating form and function." *Carcinogenesis* 28 (7): 1387-92. http://www.ncbi.nlm.nih.gov/entrez/query.fcgi?cmd=Retrieve&db=PubMed&dopt=Citation&list_uids=17434922

Kononen, J., M. Heiskanen, M. Barlund, F. Forozan, S. Ethier, J. Torhorst, G. Sauter, and O Kallioniemi. 2001. "CGH, CDNA and tissue microarray analyses of breast cancer implicate FGFR2 as a putative, but infrequent target gene for 10q26 gene amplifications in breast cancer." *Cancer Res* (In Press).

Kuang, Y., B. Siddiqui, J. Hu, M. Pun, M. Cornwell, G. Buchwalter, M. E. Hughes, N. Wagle, P. Kirschmeier, P. A. Janne, C. P. Paweletz, N. U. Lin, I. E. Krop, W. T. Barry, E. P. Winer, M. Brown, and R. Jeselsohn. 2018. "Unraveling the clinicopathological features driving the emergence of ESR1 mutations in metastatic breast cancer." *NPJ Breast Cancer* 4: 22. https://doi.org/10.1038/s41523-018-0075-5. https://www.ncbi.nlm.nih.gov/pubmed/30083595.

Kwek, S. S., R. Roy, H. Zhou, J. Climent, J. A. Martinez-Climent, J. Fridlyand, and D. G. Albertson. 2009. "Co-amplified genes at 8p12 and 11q13 in breast tumors cooperate with two major pathways in oncogenesis." *Oncogene* 28 (17): 1892-903. http://www.ncbi.nlm.nih.gov/entrez/query.fcgi?cmd=Retrieve&db=PubMed&dopt=Citation&list_uids=19330026

Lin, A., C. J. Giuliano, A. Palladino, K. M. John, C. Abramowicz, M. L. Yuan, E. L. Sausville, D. A. Lukow, L. Liu, A. R. Chait, Z. C. Galluzzo, C. Tucker, and J. M. Sheltzer. 2019. "Off-target toxicity is a common mechanism of action of cancer drugs undergoing clinical trials." *Sci Transl Med* 11 (509). https://doi.org/10.1126/scitranslmed.aaw8412. https://www.ncbi.nlm.nih.gov/pubmed/31511426.

Liu, E., A. Thor, M. He, M. Barcos, B.M. Ljung, and C. Benz. 1992. "The HER2 (c-erbB-2) Oncogene Is Frequently Amplified in Insitu Carcinomas of the Breast #651." *Oncogene* 7 (5): 1027-1032.

Lynch, T.J., D.W. Bell, R. Sordella, S. Gurubhagavatula, R.A. Okimoto, B.W. Branningan, P.L. Harris, S.M. Haserlat, J.G. Supko, F.G. Haluska, D.N. Louis, D.C. Christiani, J. Settleman, and D.A. Haber. 2004. "Activating Mutations in the Epidermal Growth Factor Receptor Underlying Responsiveness of Non-Small-Cell Lung Cancer to Gefitinib." *N Engl J Med* 350 (21).

Manohar, P. M., and N. E. Davidson. 2021. "Updates in endocrine therapy for metastatic breast cancer." *Cancer Biol Med*. https://doi.org/10.20892/j.issn.2095-3941.2021.0255. https://www.ncbi.nlm.nih.gov/pubmed/34609096.

Markopoulos, C. 2013. "Overview of the use of Oncotype DX((R)) as an additional treatment decision tool in early breast cancer." *Expert Rev Anticancer Ther* 13 (2): 179-94. https://doi.org/10.1586/era.12.174. https://www.ncbi.nlm.nih.gov/pubmed/23406559.

Marshall, C.J. 1991. "Tumor Suppressor Genes." *Cell* 64 (2): 313-326.

Marti, C., and J. I. Sanchez-Mendez. 2021. "The Present and Future of Neoadjuvant Endocrine Therapy for Breast Cancer Treatment." *Cancers (Basel)* 13 (11). https://doi.org/10.3390/cancers13112538. https://www.ncbi.nlm.nih.gov/pubmed/34064183.

Miller, B. E., F. R. Miller, and G. H. Heppner. 1984. "Assessing tumor drug sensitivity by a new in vitro assay which preserves tumor heterogeneity and subpopulation interactions." *J Cell Physiol Suppl* 3: 105-16. https://doi.org/10.1002/jcp.1041210413. https://www.ncbi.nlm.nih.gov/pubmed/6589227.

Moffa, A. B., and S. P. Ethier. 2007. "Differential signal transduction of alternatively spliced FGFR2 variants expressed in human mammary epithelial cells." *J Cell Physiol* 210 (3): 720-31. http://www.ncbi.nlm.nih.gov/entrez/query.fcgi?cmd=Retrieve&db=PubMed&dopt=Citation&list_uids=17133345.

Moffa, A. B., S. L. Tannheimer, and S. P. Ethier. 2004. "Transforming potential of alternatively spliced variants of fibroblast growth factor receptor 2 in human mammary epithelial cells." *Mol Cancer Res* 2 (11): 643-52. http://www.ncbi.nlm.nih.gov/entrez/query.fcgi?cmd=Retrieve&db=PubMed&dopt=Citation&list_uids=15561780.

Murciano-Goroff, Y. R., A. Drilon, and Z. K. Stadler. 2021. "The NCI-MATCH: A National, Collaborative Precision Oncology Trial for Diverse Tumor Histologies." *Cancer Cell* 39 (1): 22-24. https://doi.org/10.1016/j.ccell.2020.12.021. https://www.ncbi.nlm.nih.gov/pubmed/33434511.

Naffar-Abu Amara, S., H. J. Kuiken, L. M. Selfors, T. Butler, M. L. Leung, C. T. Leung, E. P. Kuhn, T. Kolarova, C. Hage, K. Ganesh, R. Panayiotou, R. Foster, B. R. Rueda, A. Aktipis, P. Spellman, T. A. Ince, J. Xiu, M. Oberley, Z. Gatalica, N. Navin, G. B. Mills, R. T. Bronson, and J. S. Brugge. 2020. "Transient commensal clonal interactions can drive tumor metastasis." *Nat Commun* 11 (1): 5799. https://doi.org/10.1038/s41467-020-19584-1. https://www.ncbi.nlm.nih.gov/pubmed/33199705.

"NCI-MATCH Sets "Benchmark of Actionability"." 2021. *Cancer Discov* 11 (1): 6-7. https://doi.org/10.1158/2159-8290.CD-NB2020-100. https://www.ncbi.nlm.nih.gov/pubmed/33168587.

Palmieri, C., T. Powles, and D. Vigushin. 2001. "Trastuzumab and breast cancer." *N Engl J Med* 345 (13): 996-997.

Papadimitriou, J.T., M. Stampfer, J. Barter, A. Lewis, M. Boshell, E.B. Lane, and I.M. Leith. 1989. "Keratin expression in human mammary cells cultured from normal and malignant tissue: relation to in vivo phenotypes and influence of medium." *J. Cell Science* 94: 403-413.

Pastan, I., and M. Gottesman. 1987. "Multiple-drug resistance in human cancer." *N Engl J Med* 316 (22): 1388-93. https://doi.org/10.1056/NEJM198705283162207. https://www.ncbi.nlm.nih.gov/pubmed/3553950.

Pejerrey, S. M., D. Dustin, J. A. Kim, G. Gu, Y. Rechoum, and S. A. W. Fuqua. 2018. "The Impact of ESR1 Mutations on the Treatment of Metastatic Breast Cancer." *Horm Cancer* 9 (4): 215-228. https://doi.org/10.1007/s12672-017-0306-5. https://www.ncbi.nlm.nih.gov/pubmed/29736566.

Penning, Trevor M. 2011. *Chemical Carcinogenesis*. edited by Trevor M. Penning: Springer.

Perez-Garcia, J., E. Munoz-Couselo, J. Soberino, F. Racca, and J. Cortes. 2018. "Targeting FGFR pathway in breast cancer." *Breast* 37: 126-133. https://doi.org/10.1016/j.breast.2017.10.014. https://www.ncbi.nlm.nih.gov/pubmed/29156384.

Periti, P., and E. Mini. 1989. "Drug resistance in cancer: an overview of the clinical aspects." *J Chemother* 1 (1): 5-9. https://doi.org/10.1080/1120009x.1989.11738856. https://www.ncbi.nlm.nih.gov/pubmed/2656931.

Poirier, Mirian C. 2018. *Carcinogens, DNA Damage and Cancer Risk*. edited by Miriam C. Poirier: World Scientific.

Prat, A., B. Adamo, M. C. Cheang, C. K. Anders, L. A. Carey, and C. M. Perou. 2013. "Molecular characterization of basal-like and non-basal-like triple-negative breast cancer." *The oncologist* 18 (2): 123-33. https://doi.org/10.1634/theoncologist.2012-0397. http://www.ncbi.nlm.nih.gov/pubmed/23404817.

Prat, A., O. Karginova, J. S. Parker, C. Fan, X. He, L. Bixby, J. C. Harrell, E. Roman, B. Adamo, M. Troester, and C. M. Perou. 2013. "Characterization of cell lines derived from breast cancers and normal mammary tissues for the study of the intrinsic molecular subtypes." *Breast cancer research and treatment* 142 (2): 237-55. https://doi.org/10.1007/s10549-013-2743-3. http://www.ncbi.nlm.nih.gov/pubmed/24162158.

Ravnan, M. C., and M. S. Matalka. 2012. "Vemurafenib in patients with BRAF V600E mutation-positive advanced melanoma." *Clin Ther* 34 (7): 1474-86. https://doi.org/10.1016/j.clinthera.2012.06.009. https://www.ncbi.nlm.nih.gov/pubmed/22742884.

Ray, M.E., Z.Q. Yang, D. Albertson, C.G. Kleer, J.G. Washburn, J.A. Macoska, and S.P. Ethier. 2004. "Genomic and Expression Analysis of the 8p11–12 Amplicon in Human Breast Cancer Cell Lines." *Cancer Res* 64 (1): 40-47.

Riely, G. J., K. A. Politi, V. A. Miller, and W. Pao. 2006. "Update on epidermal growth factor receptor mutations in non-small cell lung cancer." *Clin Cancer Res* 12 (24): 7232-41.

http://www.ncbi.nlm.nih.gov/entrez/query.fcgi?cmd=Retrieve&db=PubMed&dopt=Citation&list_uids=17189394.

Ross, D. T., and C. A. Perou. 2001. "A comparison of gene expression signatures from breast tumors and breast tissue derived cell lines." *Dis Markers* 17 (2): 99-109.

Ross, D. T., U. Scherf, M. B. Eisen, C. M. Perou, C. Rees, P. Spellman, V. Iyer, S. S. Jeffrey, M. Van de Rijn, M. Waltham, A. Pergamenschikov, J. C. Lee, D. Lashkari, D. Shalon, T. G. Myers, J. N. Weinstein, D. Botstein, and P. O. Brown. 2000. "Systematic variation in gene expression patterns in human cancer cell lines." *Nat Genet* 24 (3): 227-35. https://doi.org/10.1038/73432. http://www.ncbi.nlm.nih.gov/pubmed/10700174.

Roussel, M. F., J. R. Downing, C. W. Rettenmier, and C. J. Sherr. 1988. "A point mutation in the extracellular domain of the human CSF-1 receptor (c-fms proto-oncogene product) activates its transforming potential #356." *Cell* 55: 979-988.

Rowley, J. D. 1990. "The Philadelphia chromosome translocation. A paradigm for understanding leukemia." *Cancer* 65 (10): 2178-84. https://doi.org/10.1002/1097-0142(19900515)65:10<2178::aid-cncr2820651004>3.0.co;2-#. https://www.ncbi.nlm.nih.gov/pubmed/2189548.

Rutkovsky, A. C., E. S. Yeh, S. T. Guest, V. J. Findlay, R. C. Muise-Helmericks, K. Armeson, and S. P. Ethier. 2019. "Eukaryotic initiation factor 4E-binding protein as an oncogene in breast cancer." *BMC Cancer* 19 (1): 491. https://doi.org/10.1186/s12885-019-5667-4. https://www.ncbi.nlm.nih.gov/pubmed/31122207.

Santarius, T., J. Shipley, D. Brewer, M. R. Stratton, and C. S. Cooper. 2010. "A census of amplified and overexpressed human cancer genes." *Nat Rev Cancer* 10 (1): 59-64. https://doi.org/10.1038/nrc2771. http://www.ncbi.nlm.nih.gov/pubmed/20029424.

Sekiya T, Prassolov VS, Fushimi M, and Nishimura S. 1985. "Transforming activity of the c-Ha-ras oncogene having two point mutations in codons 12 and 61." *Jpn J Cancer Res* 76 (9): 851-5.

Sflomos, G., L. Battista, P. Aouad, F. De Martino, V. Scabia, A. Stravodimou, A. Ayyanan, A. Ifticene-Treboux, Rls, P. Bucher, M.

Fiche, G. Ambrosini, and C. Brisken. 2021. "Intraductal xenografts show lobular carcinoma cells rely on their own extracellular matrix and LOXL1." *EMBO Mol Med* 13 (3): e13180. https://doi.org/10.15252/emmm.202013180. https://www.ncbi.nlm.nih.gov/pubmed/33616307.

Sharma, A., S. R. Shah, H. Illum, and J. Dowell. 2012. "Vemurafenib: targeted inhibition of mutated BRAF for treatment of advanced melanoma and its potential in other malignancies." *Drugs* 72 (17): 2207-22. https://doi.org/10.2165/11640870-000000000-00000. https://www.ncbi.nlm.nih.gov/pubmed/23116250.

Shekhar, M. P., I. Kato, P. Nangia-Makker, and L. Tait. 2013. "Comedo-DCIS is a precursor lesion for basal-like breast carcinoma: identification of a novel p63/Her2/neu expressing subgroup." *Oncotarget* 4 (2): 231-41. https://doi.org/10.18632/oncotarget.818. https://www.ncbi.nlm.nih.gov/pubmed/23548208.

Shepherd, F. A., J. Rodrigues Pereira, T. Ciuleanu, E. H. Tan, V. Hirsh, S. Thongprasert, D. Campos, S. Maoleekoonpiroj, M. Smylie, R. Martins, M. van Kooten, M. Dediu, B. Findlay, D. Tu, D. Johnston, A. Bezjak, G. Clark, P. Santabarbara, and L. Seymour. 2005. "Erlotinib in previously treated non-small-cell lung cancer." *N Engl J Med* 353 (2): 123-32. http://www.ncbi.nlm.nih.gov/entrez/query.fcgi?cmd=Retrieve&db=PubMed&dopt=Citation&list_uids=16014882.

Skloot, Rebecca. 2011. *The immortal life of Henrietta Lacks*. Crown.

Slamon, D., B. Leyland-Jones, S. Shak, V. Paton, A. Bajamonde, T. Fleming, W. Eirmann, J. Wolter, J. Baselga, and L. Norton. 1998. "Addition of Herceptin (humanized anti-HER2 antibody) to first line chemotherapy for HER2 overexpressing metastatic breast cancer markedly increases anticancer activity: a randomized, multinational controlled Phase III trial. #1806." *Proceedings of ASCO* 377 (17): 98a.

Smith, Y. E., G. Wang, C. L. Flynn, S. F. Madden, O. MacEneaney, R. G. B. Cruz, C. E. Richards, H. Jahns, M. Brennan, M. Cremona, B. T. Hennessy, K. Sheehan, A. Casucci, F. A. Sani, L. Hudson, J. Fay, S. H. Vellanki, S. O'Flaherty, M. Devocelle, A. D. K. Hill, K. Brennan, S. Sukumar, and A. M. Hopkins. 2022. "Functional Antagonism of Junctional Adhesion Molecule-A (JAM-A), Overexpressed in Breast Ductal Carcinoma In Situ (DCIS), Reduces HER2-Positive Tumor Progression." *Cancers (Basel)* 14 (5). https://doi.org/10.3390/cancers14051303. https://www.ncbi.nlm.nih.gov/pubmed/35267611.

Soule, H. D., J. Vazguez, A. Long, S Albert, and M Brennan. 1973. "A human cell line from a pleural effusion derived from a breast carcinoma." *J. Natl. Cancer. Inst.* 51: 1409-1416.

Soule, H.D., T.M. Malony, S.R. Wolman, W.D. Peterson, R. Brenz, C.M. McGrath, J. Russo, R.J. Pauley, R.F. Jones, and S.C. Brooks. 1990.

"Isolation and characterization of a spontaneously immortalized human breast epithelial cell line, MCF-10." *Cancer Res.* 50 (18): 6075-6086.

Speers, C., and L. J. Pierce. 2016. "Postoperative Radiotherapy After Breast-Conserving Surgery for Early-Stage Breast Cancer: A Review." *JAMA Oncol* 2 (8): 1075-82. https://doi.org/10.1001/jamaoncol.2015.5805. https://www.ncbi.nlm.nih.gov/pubmed/27243924.

Stampfer, M.R., R.C. Hallowes, and A.J. Hackett. 1980. "Growth of normal human mammary epithelial cells in culture." *In Vitro* 16: 415-425.

Streicher, K. L., Z. Q. Yang, S. Draghici, and S. P. Ethier. 2007. "Transforming function of the LSM1 oncogene in human breast cancers with the 8p11-12 amplicon." *Oncogene* 26 (14): 2104-14. http://www.ncbi.nlm.nih.gov/entrez/query.fcgi?cmd=Retrieve&db=PubMed&dopt=Citation&list_uids=17001308.

Suo, Z. , B. Risberg, M.G. Kalsson, K. Willman, A. Tierens, E. Skovlund, and J.M. Nesland. 2002. "EGFR family expression in breast carcinomas. c-erbB-2 and c-erbB-4 receptors have different effects on survial." *J Pathol* 196 (1): 17-25.

Swain, S. M., J. Baselga, S. B. Kim, J. Ro, V. Semiglazov, M. Campone, E. Ciruelos, J. M. Ferrero, A. Schneeweiss, S. Heeson, E. Clark, G. Ross, M. C. Benyunes, J. Cortes, and Cleopatra Study Group. 2015. "Pertuzumab, trastuzumab, and docetaxel in HER2-positive metastatic breast cancer." *N Engl J Med* 372 (8): 724-34. https://doi.org/10.1056/NEJMoa1413513. http://www.ncbi.nlm.nih.gov/pubmed/25693012.

Tannheimer, S. L., A. Rehemtulla, and S. P. Ethier. 2000. "Characterization of fibroblast growth factor receptor 2 overexpression in the human breast cancer cell line SUM-52PE." *Breast Cancer Res* 2 (4): 311-20. http://www.ncbi.nlm.nih.gov/entrez/query.fcgi?cmd=Retrieve&db=PubMed&dopt=Citation&list_uids=11056689.

Trosko, J. E., and R. J. Ruch. 1998. "Cell-cell communication in carcinogenesis." *Front Biosci* 3: d208-36. https://doi.org/10.2741/a275. https://www.ncbi.nlm.nih.gov/pubmed/9458335.

Tsao, M. S., A. Sakurada, J. C. Cutz, C. Q. Zhu, S. Kamel-Reid, J. Squire, I. Lorimer, T. Zhang, N. Liu, M. Daneshmand, P. Marrano, G. da Cunha Santos, A. Lagarde, F. Richardson, L. Seymour, M. Whitehead, K. Ding, J. Pater, and F. A. Shepherd. 2005. "Erlotinib in lung cancer - molecular and clinical predictors of outcome." *N Engl J Med* 353 (2): 133-44.

http://www.ncbi.nlm.nih.gov/entrez/query.fcgi?cmd=Retrieve&db=PubMed&dopt=Citation&list_uids=16014883.

Tsherniak, A., F. Vazquez, P. G. Montgomery, B. A. Weir, G. Kryukov, G. S. Cowley, S. Gill, W. F. Harrington, S. Pantel, J. M. Krill-Burger, R. M. Meyers, L. Ali, A. Goodale, Y. Lee, G. Jiang, J. Hsiao, W. F. J. Gerath, S. Howell, E. Merkel, M. Ghandi, L. A. Garraway, D. E. Root, T. R. Golub, J. S. Boehm, and W. C. Hahn. 2017. "Defining a Cancer Dependency Map." *Cell* 170 (3): 564-576 e16. https://doi.org/10.1016/j.cell.2017.06.010. https://www.ncbi.nlm.nih.gov/pubmed/28753430.

Turner-Ivey, B., S. T. Guest, J. C. Irish, C. S. Kappler, E. Garrett-Mayer, R. C. Wilson, and S. P. Ethier. 2014. "KAT6A, a chromatin modifier from the 8p11-p12 amplicon is a candidate oncogene in luminal breast cancer." *Neoplasia* 16 (8): 644-55. https://doi.org/10.1016/j.neo.2014.07.007. http://www.ncbi.nlm.nih.gov/pubmed/25220592.

Turner-Ivey, B., E. L. Smith, A. C. Rutkovsky, L. S. Spruill, J. N. Mills, and S. P. Ethier. 2017. "Development of mammary hyperplasia, dysplasia, and invasive ductal carcinoma in transgenic mice expressing the 8p11 amplicon oncogene NSD3." *Breast Cancer Res Treat* 164 (2): 349-358. https://doi.org/10.1007/s10549-017-4258-9. https://www.ncbi.nlm.nih.gov/pubmed/28484924.

Upton, Arthur C. 1986. *Radiation Carcinogenesis*. Elsevier Science Ltd.

Wang, G., G. Liu, X. Wang, S. Sethi, R. Ali-Fehmi, J. Abrams, Z. Zheng, K. Zhang, S. Ethier, and Z. Q. Yang. 2012. "ERLIN2 promotes breast cancer cell survival by modulating endoplasmic reticulum stress pathways." *BMC cancer* 12: 225. https://doi.org/10.1186/1471-2407-12-225. http://www.ncbi.nlm.nih.gov/pubmed/22681620.

Wang, T., K. Birsoy, N. W. Hughes, K. M. Krupczak, Y. Post, J. J. Wei, E. S. Lander, and D. M. Sabatini. 2015. "Identification and characterization of essential genes in the human genome." *Science* 350 (6264): 1096-101. https://doi.org/10.1126/science.aac7041. https://www.ncbi.nlm.nih.gov/pubmed/26472758.

Wang, T., E. S. Lander, and D. M. Sabatini. 2016. "Viral Packaging and Cell Culture for CRISPR-Based Screens." *Cold Spring Harb Protoc* 2016 (3): pdb prot090811. https://doi.org/10.1101/pdb.prot090811. https://www.ncbi.nlm.nih.gov/pubmed/26933250.

Wang, T., J. J. Wei, D. M. Sabatini, and E. S. Lander. 2014. "Genetic screens in human cells using the CRISPR-Cas9 system." *Science* 343 (6166): 80-4. https://doi.org/10.1126/science.1246981. https://www.ncbi.nlm.nih.gov/pubmed/24336569.

Weinberg, R. 1991. "Tumor suppressor genes." *Science* 254 (5035): 1138-1146.

Weinstein, B. 1987. "Growth Factors, Oncogenes, and multistage carcinogenesis." *J. Cell. Biochem.* 33: 213-224.

Weinstein, I. B., M. Begemann, P. Zhou, E. K. Han, A. Sgambato, Y. Doki, N. Arber, M. Ciaparrone, and H. Yamamoto. 1997. "Disorders in cell circuitry associated with multistage carcinogenesis: exploitable targets for cancer prevention and therapy." *Clin Cancer Res* 3 (12 Pt 2): 2696-702. http://www.ncbi.nlm.nih.gov/pubmed/10068276.

Weinstein, I. B., and A. Joe. 2008. "Oncogene addiction." *Cancer Res* 68 (9): 3077-80; discussion 3080. https://doi.org/10.1158/0008-5472.CAN-07-3293. http://www.ncbi.nlm.nih.gov/pubmed/18451130.

Weinstein, I. B., and A. K. Joe. 2006. "Mechanisms of disease: Oncogene addiction--a rationale for molecular targeting in cancer therapy." *Nat Clin Pract Oncol* 3 (8): 448-57. https://doi.org/10.1038/ncponc0558. http://www.ncbi.nlm.nih.gov/pubmed/16894390.

Yang, Z. Q., D. Albertson, and S. P. Ethier. 2004. "Genomic organization of the 8p11-p12 amplicon in three breast cancer cell lines." *Cancer Genet Cytogenet* 155 (1): 57-62. http://www.ncbi.nlm.nih.gov/entrez/query.fcgi?cmd=Retrieve&db=PubMed&dopt=Citation&list_uids=15527903.

Yang, Z. Q., G. Liu, A. Bollig-Fischer, C. N. Giroux, and S. P. Ethier. 2010. "Transforming properties of 8p11-12 amplified genes in human breast cancer." *Cancer Res* 70 (21): 8487-97. https://doi.org/10.1158/0008-5472.CAN-10-1013. http://www.ncbi.nlm.nih.gov/pubmed/20940404.

Yang, Z. Q., G. Liu, A. Bollig-Fischer, R. Haddad, A. L. Tarca, and S. P. Ethier. 2009. "Methylation-associated silencing of SFRP1 with an 8p11-12 amplification inhibits canonical and non-canonical WNT pathways in breast cancers." *Int J Cancer* 125 (7): 1613-21. http://www.ncbi.nlm.nih.gov/entrez/query.fcgi?cmd=Retrieve&db=PubMed&dopt=Citation&list_uids=19569235

Yang, Z. Q., K. L. Streicher, M. E. Ray, J. Abrams, and S. P. Ethier. 2006. "Multiple interacting oncogenes on the 8p11-p12 amplicon in human breast cancer." *Cancer Res* 66 (24): 11632-43. http://www.ncbi.nlm.nih.gov/entrez/query.fcgi?cmd=Retrieve&db=PubMed&dopt=Citation&list_uids=17178857.

Zhang, K., R. Hong, F. Xu, W. Xia, L. Kaping, G. Qin, Q. Zheng, Q. Lu, Y. X. Shi, Z. Y. Yuan, and S. Wang. 2018. "Clinical value of circulating ESR1 mutations for patients with metastatic breast cancer: a meta-analysis." *Cancer Manag Res* 10: 2573-2580.

https://doi.org/10.2147/CMAR.S173193.
https://www.ncbi.nlm.nih.gov/pubmed/30147360.

INDEX